3/17/06

Dear Maxanes

FOOD SWINGS

Control your
Food swings
+ Be well

BARNET MELTZER, M.D.

WITH SIOBHAN MCGOWAN

FOOD SWINGS

MARLOWE & COMPANY
NEW YORK

Published by

Marlowe & Company

An Imprint of Avalon Publishing Group Incorporated

841 Broadway, 4th Floor

New York, NY 10003

Food Swings: *Make the Life-Changing Connection Between the Foods You Eat and Your Emotional Health and Well-Being*

The information in this book is intended to help readers make informed decisions about their health and the health of their loved ones. It is not intended to be a substitute for treatment by or the advice and care of a professional health care provider. While the author and publisher have endeavored to ensure that the information presented is accurate and up-to-date, they are not responsible for adverse effects or consequences sustained by any person using this book.

Library of Congress Cataloging-in-Publication Data

Meltzer, Barnet.

Food swings : making the life changing connection between the food you eat and your emotional well-being / by Barnet G. Meltzer.

p. cm.

ISBN 1-56924-682-3

1. Mental Health—Nutritional aspects. 2. Nutrition. I. Title.

RC455.4.N8 M44 1999

613.2—dc21

99-044602

9 8 7 6 5 4 3 2 1

DESIGNED BY PAULINE NEUWIRTH, NEUWIRTH & ASSOCIATES, INC.

Distributed by Publishers Group West

Printed in the United States of America

CONTENTS

CONTENTS

CONTENTS

CONTENTS

CONTENTS

PREFACE

Food Swings **tells** the fascinating story of how the foods you eat influence how you feel. Does that sound basic? In fact, it is. But *Food Swings* also gets to the heart of what it takes for lifelong health and happiness. We all have to eat—in fact, we all eat several times a day, every day, day in and day out. Yet amazingly, many of us simply never take the time to slow down enough to become aware of the relationship between the foods we eat and our moods—our *food swings*, as I like to call them. What could be more basic than paying attention to this?

In 1972, I became the first medical doctor to begin practicing preventive medicine in Southern California, where I continue to practice today, nearly thirty years later. Over the past three decades, I have interviewed some 35,000 patients in my role as their primary care preventive medical specialist. I often tell my patients two things: First, and most importantly, "The least costly illness is the one that never occurs. You've got to learn to take care of yourself so you can get to it before it gets to you." And second, I tell my patients that I am a "thrivologist." I am there to help them to thrive and to free themselves not only from ill health, but also, and as importantly, from the emotional dysfunction that causes fatigue, depression, anxiety, weight gain, and a loss of sexual vitality. This emotional distress may be keeping them from being the best person they can be.

Over the years I have asked every single one of my patients to rate their energy level from one to ten, with ten, of course, being the top of the line. What do you think they say? Most of my patients put their energy level somewhere in the four to seven range. When I question them as to whether it is a steady four or a steady seven, from morning until the end of the day, they invariably answer that their energy level drops in midday or by late afternoon, and then they may rally after dinner and then crash.

Anything less than a consistent nine or ten will have a negative impact on the quality of your life. I tell them they have a clear choice. They can choose to be well. This is where *Food Swings* comes in. *Food Swings* will teach you which foods make you feel energetic and bold and which foods will make you feel sleepy, tired, or anxious. But *Food Swings* will also introduce you to your own experiential—and experimental learning process. It will guide you by tuning you into your own personality and metabolic individuality so that you can choose foods that make you feel good all day long, all life long.

Like many of my patients, you may have been waiting your whole life to understand how you can be an emotional winner—how you can live your dream and consistently be happy, loving, emotionally engaged, physically healthy, soulful, and successful. My purpose in writing *Food Swings* is to provide you with information and strategies that will serve you every time you decide to eat—day in and day out—lessons that will help you to learn to take care of yourself, physically and emotionally, by choosing the foods that are going to be best for you.

Thanks for coming along on this ride with me. I look forward to hearing your *Food Swings* success stories.

INTRODUCTION

How do you feel at the end of the day? Down and burnt out? Moody? Hungry? Have you ever wondered why you're sluggish and drowsy soon after eating? I promise that by the time you finish *Food Swings*, you'll understand the connection between the foods you eat and your emotional, physical, and psychological health and well-being.

Your eating habits are the action. Food swings—the moods and behaviors set in motion by the meals you eat—are the reaction. Food swings are the changes that take place in your attitude and energy level from consuming food and drink. These swings can make or break you, bolster your health or bring it down, reign you in or stress you out. Food swings illustrate how your choice of foods either elevates or deflates your emotions.

What is the key to good nutrition? If you answered "a healthy diet," you're only partially right. Good nutrition is not just about broccoli, carrots, and "an apple a day." It also involves your eating habits. And there's a lot more to these habits than food itself.

Not only what you eat, but when, where, how, *how much*, and, perhaps most important, *why* you eat all influence your dietary state. What specific triggers set you off on a binge? Think about it, and you'll find that your eating habits express much more about you than just your favorite flavor of ice cream.

STRESS PLAYS HAVOC WITH YOUR EATING HABITS

Healthy eating habits put you in a good mood. To establish healthy eating habits, you'll need a balanced emotional life. When you are under stress you don't eat right and your eating habits have a tendency to fall apart. You start looking for a mood change and food might just be your answer. Unfortunately, stress is widespread, and it wreaks havoc on both emotions and, by extension, behavior. The firmest New Year resolutions tend to fall apart under the pressure of stress, and it's all too easy to turn to food for comfort. After a rotten day at work, what's your particular crutch? Beer? Pizza? Chocolate chip cookies?

Junk food provides a temporary, false improvement in mood, but its long-term effects are just the opposite. You crash after consuming too much sugar. Too many carbs send you to bed. Alcohol depresses. Your momentary high is followed by a debilitating low which only increases the stress—on your metabolism, your mentality, and your emotions. A poor diet doesn't counter stress. It compounds it.

For the past several years, we have been experiencing an explosion of interest in clinical nutrition. More and more research contributes to the theories that food contains medicinal properties—that healthy food heals. Everyday, scientists discover something new about the wonders of fresh fruits, vegetables, grains, and legumes. Different ingredients and nutrients are shown to reduce the risks of cancer, heart disease, arthritis, stroke, multiple sclerosis, Alzheimer's, and other debilitating, seemingly incurable, degenerative illnesses.

And yet, a puzzling paradox exists. At a time when we are more knowledgeable than ever about the positive impact of good nutrition, we are, as a society, sicker than ever. Frankly, our eating habits are out of control. In spite of the media focus on fitness and thinness, Americans are plagued by an increase in obesity, an increase in chronic disease, and a decline in the quality of life. Our fast-paced, hi-tech lifestyle has left us computer literate but emotionally illiterate and nutritionally out of focus. We're stressed, confused, tense, tired, restless. We're fat, or anorexic, or bulimic, or carb-or protein-addicted.

Isn't it ironic that, simultaneous to the rebirth of interest in organic produce and physical health, the fast-food industry is thriving? Meat and dairy industries are going strong. Sweets, fats, and party-food favorites dominate the airwaves and tyrannize TV. Supermarkets are stocked with artificial food. The **S**tandard **A**merican **D**iet is a s-a-d excuse for nutrition.

We know so much, but we choose food as if we know nothing. We eagerly gather information, but are loath to apply it. Why is this? That's the complex question I aim to answer with this book. I want you to make the connection between stress levels, repressed emotions, and poor eating habits.

STRESS DICTATES YOUR EATING HABITS

Negative, or dysfunctional, food swings are synonymous with bad eating habits. Stress triggers such habits: overeating, bingeing, compulsive snacking, late-night indulgences, sweet teeth, and so on. It's the driving force behind cravings and addictions, and it sets into motion a SAD, self-abusive cycle: stress leads to poor food choices; poor food choices lead to lethargy, depression, ill health—in other words, more stress.

The majority of dysfunctional food swings are responses to emotional stress. People who are overworked, love-starved, or lonely turn to food for comfort. And yet, the chemical side effects of poor food choices only contribute to the overall tension.

EAT YOURSELF HAPPY

Positive, or healthy, food swings synchronize nutritious foods with smart habits— habits like undereating for energy and knowing when enough is enough. Positive food swings energize and inspire. They increase sexual appeal and performance. They enable you to work harder and smarter. They do more than just build good behavior: They build self-confidence, character, willpower, discipline, esteem.

Healthy food swings are the missing link between diet and emotions. They reach deep down inside and improve our ability to cope with the curveballs life's constantly throwing our way. Dysfunctional food swings, on the other hand, will inevitably do us in. They will plague anyone who continues to eat the wrong kinds and amounts of food in response to stress.

Food Swings will teach you to choose foods and create the eating habits that protect mind, body, and soul from the symptoms of stress—premature aging and disease. It outlines what foods reduce stress, increase energy, combat depression, and heighten sexuality. It will tell you how to transcend the temptations.

A THREE-PRONGED APPROACH

Food Swings is divided into three separate-but-equal sections. Part 1, "Stress and Your Eating Habits," gets to the root of your mommy-daddy diet. It defines emotional tension and describes the three degrees of metabolic burnout. In it, I reveal the Golden Rules for Smart Eating, foolproof formulas for conquering stress and achieving high-performance nutrition, and the Top Ten Stress-Inducing Foods. I also explain in practical terms "antioxidants," which are being highly touted for their various benefits.

Part 2, "Prevent Dysfunctional Food Swings and Take Control of Your Diet," classifies eight of the most common dysfunctional food swings, explores the emerging field of emoto-nutrition, and offers an assortment of smart food choices to ward off depression and anxiety, bolster energy levels, and even improve your love life.

Part 3, "Food Personalities," could be a book unto itself. Quaint as it may sound, each food actually has its own character, whether it's the take-charge power of spinach, the down-to-earth nature of potatoes, or the succulent sensuality of ripe tomatoes. Through five categories—fruits, vegetables, legumes, grains, and nuts and seeds—Part 3 describes how different foods influence different dispositions, moods, and attitudes. From apples to zucchini, you'll discover not only the therapeutic properties of foods, but also their distinct identities. And with that knowledge, you can orchestrate your diet to alter your personality—for the better, of course!

YOUR NUTRITIONAL COACH

My job, as I see it, is to fill your head with nutritional common sense. I want to train you to achieve your maximum nutritional potential through smart food choices, sound eating habits, and positive food swings. Like any goal, it will require some discipline: a daily Sunrise Cleanse and Sunset Recharge, for example. But the payoffs are great. Stick with me, and you'll learn:

- How to side-step high stress levels
- How to conquer food addiction
- How to overcome overeating
- How to lose weight permanently
- How to prevent stress-related dysfunctional food swings
- How to reduce and eliminate dysfunctional eating habits
- How to avoid mood swings
- How to select the foods that are best for you

I believe you'll find it fascinating how eating habits influence emotional well-being. I know that, in my many years as an MD and an advocate of preventive medicine, I have been astonished by the power of whole foods. Share my amazement, and profit from my experience. Improve your habits, reduce stress, strengthen your immune system, and learn to live fully. Ready? Let's go!

PART 1

STRESS AND YOUR EATING HABITS:

YOU ARE HOW YOU EAT

THERE'S A conspiracy at work. It wants you to spend your money on fast, convenient food that will pump your bloodstream and systems with sugar, salt, and fat. In your adult life, this conspiracy takes the form of advertising and big business, but the seeds were planted in your subconscious when you were just a kid. That's when you learned about the emotional aspects of food and developed your particular diet based on your particular family and its dining rituals. Check out the Top Ten Anti-Nutrients, in Chapter 4, and see how many of your childhood favorites make the list.

The problem is, the junk-food conspiracy places its profits over your health, so it's time to save yourself—before the Standard American Diet (SAD) diet and emotional tension take you by the seat of your ever-expanding pants and kick you down the three-step staircase of metabolic burnout. But don't fear, help is here—in the form of my proven formulas and the Golden Rules of Eating.

CHAPTER 1

YOUR EATING HABITS
AND YOUR EMOTIONS

Although we don't always think of it as such, diet is one of the most emotional issues in modern life—as emotional, in fact, as sex, religion, and politics. Today, many of us are self-aware enough to know that how we feel—our mood swings—affects what we eat, but we often overlook the other half of the equation. Like any other relationship, the connection between food and feelings is a two-way street: What we eat—our food swings—affects how we feel. Emotional stress adversely influences our eating habits, and our negative eating habits, in turn, wreak havoc with our emotions. It's a vicious cycle—the dietary equivalent of a dog chasing its own tail.

It's time for a détente. To strike a balance between emotions and eating habits is a sound, soulful aim. When your emotional and nutritional powers work together, vibrant health follows. *Food Swings* will give you the tools to achieve this equilibrium.

But what good are tools if you don't know how to use them? Before you can fix a problem, you have to understand it. Moods and food choices touch each other in myriad ways. People look to their meals for more than just nutritional input—sadly, that's sometimes the last consideration, if it's thought of at all. No, instead, we eat for comfort, or companionship, or to satisfy a craving. We focus on all the social aspects of eating: the most convenient meals to buy, the current culinary trends, the hottest restaurants. It's human nature—and it's unhealthy.

Think about your favorite foods. They have an emotional appeal, even a physical attraction, don't they? Undoubtedly, your favorites have a special taste, look, and smell. You profess your undying devotion to chocolate, French fries, sirloin steak. You cannot resist their smell, taste, charm. You lick your fingers and smack your lips. Munching away on preferred foods is one of life's greatest pleasures. Pasta stuffed with cheese and swimming in sauce, salty tortilla chips dipped in salsa, submarine sandwiches stacked with deli meats, cartons of Chinese take-out, birthday cake topped with ice cream scoops and garnished with candy bits and cookie crumbles—if loving them is wrong, why does it feel so right? Our lives revolve around food. We live to eat. Events big and small, good and bad, are commemorated with special meals—breakfast in bed on Mother's Day, dinner out to celebrate a promotion, a pint of ice cream when the romance ends. Remember McDonald's™ old slogan? "You deserve a break today." We emotionally reward ourselves with food, instead of choosing ingredients for their high-octane nutritive value and biological benefits.

The short-term satisfaction that comes from indulging in our favorite foods, however, can't compare with the long-term effects of proper eating. That's no secret. A wholesome diet leads to positive food swings and optimum health. Quality eating habits are the building blocks of preventive medicine. They fuel a high-performance lifestyle, and the discipline they demand strengthens body, mind, and spirit. Quality eating habits actually equip you to deal constructively with stress and foster an emotional climate conducive to happiness.

YOUR EATING HABITS DON'T LIE

Your eating habits tell the story. What, when, where, why, and how you eat reveal the relationship between your diet and your emotions. The foods you select, the quantity you consume, the time you dine, and the speed with which you wash it down all define your eating habits. More subtle factors include your appetite, posture, mood, and mental attitude. In fact, your mood often determines whether or not you're hungry. A clear mind and relaxed body know how much food is enough.

Eating well has more to do with positive habits than informed thinking. That's because eating well involves making the right choices, and not just eating the right foods. It's as much behavioral as intellectual: If you know vegetables are good for you but you don't eat them, then what good is that knowledge?

We all want to have an interesting, impassioned, fulfilling relationship with our food. Enjoyment in eating is one of our most basic instincts. But if it feels good to eat, it feels even better to eat right. The key to wholesome food swings can be summarized in a single sentence: **Undereating high-quality foods at the right time in a relaxed manner forms the foundation for optimum health.**

Right time, relaxed manner. Got it?

It's all too common to be attached to foods that ultimately are damaging. They appeal to our senses. Frankly, there's a sexual, physical component to most snacks—we eat them hand to mouth. Beyond that, we associate certain foods with powerful memories, and eat to relive them. Do some soul-searching and figure out the meanings you've subconsciously assigned to favorite foods.

THE MOMMY-DADDY DIET

The foods you grew up with form your first, and often only, diet—your base diet, the meals you return to week after week. I sometimes refer to it as the Mommy-Daddy diet. You're familiar with these foods—they're like childhood friends. They remind you of your youth, and of time spent with siblings, parents, and relatives. Little did you know at eleven years old that you were already being programmed for a particular pathology of eating that would come to dominate your adult life. And yet, looking back, didn't your favorite foods relate to a reward system? Didn't parents treat you with ice cream or pizza if you'd behaved well? Didn't you get to choose the restaurant on your birthday?

Ours is also the culture of instant gratification. Instead of considering how we'll feel two hours after downing that bacon cheeseburger, we can only think of now, of how good that first bite is going to taste. In America, we swear by the motto "Work Hard, Play Hard"—and, by extension, "Party Hardy." Food is a recreational drug. For heaven's sake, we're the home of the free, land of the hot-dog eating contest! Of course, eating is a social activity, and can be a wonderful way to relax with others. But problems result when eating becomes the focus of a get-together, and not just a way to enhance it. Equally sad, overeating often occurs when you're alone—to remind you of when you did have a large, loving group around you. Mommy-daddy foods become a major source of security in a lonely, scary world.

We've been conditioned to use food as an emotional reward system. We've been trained to release pent-up sexual energy and professional frustrations through food. We use it as a coping mechanism and to comfort ourselves. We've been unwilling guinea pigs, brainwashed into such destructive behavior. Now our challenge is to break the cycle.

CONSTANT COMPANION

Over-attachment to your mommy-daddy diet sets the stage for negative food swings. Eating habits become a crutch: When you're hurt, depressed, or disappointed, you reach for your favorite snacks, sweets, and sandwiches. When friends, family, and spouse let you down, food's a constant companion. There you sit, TV remote in one hand, potato chips in the other, avoiding all the problems in your life. After a while, you become so mesmerized by your chosen foods that you may as well be having a love affair with them. You can't wait to see them, you rush home after a hard day to greet them, you conduct clandestine rendezvous out in the garage or locked behind the bathroom door. Whenever they're not readily available, you feel irritated, angry, deprived.

As you get to know your own emotional profile and the effect it has on your eating habits, you'll discover the simple truth: Dietary patterns help you to escape the conflicts in your life. Put another way, appetite is heavily influenced by mood. When you're stressed, you look to food for emotional comfort. Rather than squarely facing your personal hurdles and making the appropriate adjustments, you numb the pain by filling your stomach.

Are you using your diet as a pacifier? Early warning signs that your emotional register is off-kilter include anxiety, depression, and irritability. But have no fear. Because eating habits and emotional reactions are interrelated, you can cure yourself. Whole foods and wholesome habits combine to create a powerful weapon against the enemy—stress. High-performance nutrition balances your brain chemistry, equalizing your emotions. Nutritious meals keep you in a good mood, and the calm that results encourages you to continue to make sound, conscientious food choices.

FEELINGS VS. EMOTIONS

If appetite, like mood, is emotionally driven, then the first step toward establishing healthy food swings involves establishing healthy eating habits. To do this, you must become familiar with your feelings and your emotions. Most of us don't think to make a distinction between the two, but understanding the difference helps us to advance to higher levels of emotional fitness.

Feelings are an inside job. They're about sensations, impressions, experiences of heart and soul. You know what it feels like to give and receive warmth and affection. You know when you're in love (when you're not sure, you're probably not!). Feelings rate in levels: okay, great, orgasmic. You know when you feel bad, you know when you feel good. You know that stress does not feel good.

Emotions are the expression of these feelings. Like the plucked strings of a guitar, they vibrate with their designated note. When you feel bad, you cry, sulk, shout. When you feel good, you smile, sing, laugh. Across the board, there's a reactive element to emotions. You may describe someone as "emotional" when she's excited, agitated, angry, upset.

The stronger the feelings, the stronger the emotions. Feelings of trust and affection encourage loving gestures. Energetic, enthusiastic feelings move you to passion and playfulness. Joyousness puts a smile on your face and a spring in your step. Conversely, feelings of anger, fear, and frustration can lead to more negative outbursts.

Before you can alter your eating habits, you have to be attuned to your feelings, good and bad. Most of us use food as a way to detach from our feelings. The destructive eating habits that occur as a consequence cause negative food swings.

In spite of the advances in technology and telecommunication, the majority of people—particularly those over the age of thirty—are disconnected, and drowning in an ocean of confusion. Public schools focus on reading, writing, and arithmetic. Institutions of higher education emphasize mental development at the expense of emotional maturity. And while there's much to be said for academic acuity, the smarter we get, the broader the gap between our intellect and our emotions. It's a sign of the times that the higher our IQ, or Intelligence Quotient, the lower our EQ, or Emotional Quotient.

It's not easy to shut off our feelings—but somehow we manage to do it. We've learned by watching our parents, and we do our best to carry on the tradition. There's a price to pay for all this repression: emotional stress. In some form or other, emotions have to find an escape, and if they can't be released in an open, positive way, then they'll find a more malignant manner to work through our system.

YOU NEED AN EMOTIONAL COMPASS

If you're not comfortable and capable of embracing your feelings, you lack an emotional compass. If you were lost in the wilderness, you'd need a compass to find your way back to civilization. The same metaphor holds true for our inner landscape. You need an emotional compass to navigate your way out of the morass of your sublimated feelings.

Our modern-day merry-go-round lifestyle can turn into a ceaseless spinning wheel of stress. In all the confusion, it's easy to lose perspective of our eating habits. By recording what you eat, when you eat, and how often you eat, you can get a grasp of your ingrained, unconscious eating patterns. Tracking your own dietary inventory will enable you to take charge of your habits, instead of allowing them to control you.

Most of us aren't even aware of how often we obsess about food. We are a culture with food on the brain. The multibillion-dollar fast-food industry profits daily from this fact: The average American eats at a fast-food outlet between fifteen and twenty times a month. The terminology—"fast" food—emphasizes the convenience of these meals, the precious time saved. But to reverse the tide of obesity that has taken over the country, we need to switch our attention to "slow" food and reevaluate our priorities. Wholesome, high-quality slow food nourishes us to wellness.

SIZE UP YOUR EMOTIONAL CONNECTION TO YOUR DIET

Who wants to analyze their feelings while eating? Who knows what ugly creatures might crawl out from under that rock? If ignorance is bliss, then knowledge is power. The truth hurts, but it will help you to understand, for example, why it's more appealing to scarf down a pizza than to prepare a fresh meal, or what destructive effects additives, preservatives, and carcinogens can have on your body. Self-assessment and making time to keep track of your eating habits is your initial call to action.

If you want to lose weight, look good, and feel great, you need to understand your connection to your favorite foods, as well as the emotional and physical costs of your eating habits. On the following chart, rate your mood and degree of hunger each time you eat for the next several days. The results will give you a handy overview of your present dietary patterns. Remember, you can't fix a problem until you know it exists. Self-assessment leads to self-correction. If you don't recognize it, a bad eating habit can creep up on you at any time and sabotage your best intentions.

EATING HABITS SURVEY

In the appropriate square mark the time of day you eat, including snacks. In the upper half of the square, rate your feelings. In the lower half, rate your appetite according to your perceived degree of hunger. For example S/3 if you're feeling extremely hungry and stressed, or H/O if you're happy and not hungry at all.

FEELINGS (ABBREVIATE)

(H)	Happy
(S)	Stressed
(A)	Anxious
(C)	Content
(E)	Emotionally Upset
(R)	Relaxed
(D)	Depressed

HUNGER

0 None
1 Mild Hunger
2 Moderate
3 Extreme

	5-6AM	6-7AM	7-8AM	8-9AM	9-10AM	10-11AM	11-12PM	12-1PM	1-2PM	2-3PM	3-4PM	4-5PM	5-6PM	6-7PM	8-9PM	9-10PM	10-11PM	11-12PM	12-1AM	1-2AM	2-3AM	3-4AM	4-5AM	Bowel Movements	Time Spent Eating
DAY 1																									
DAY 2																									
DAY 3																									
DAY 4																									
DAY 5																									

In the following spaces, make some notes on what you have learned from this exercise. What connection can you see between your emotions and your eating habits? What are you usually feeling when you're hungry? How does your stress level influence your eating habits?

As human beings, we have to eat. There's no quitting cold turkey, the way we might with, for example, cigarettes or alcohol. A personal involvement with your diet is inescapable, so why not strive to make the relationship a positive, nurturing one? Love and respect your diet the way you would a best friend. It will reward you with boundless energy and positive mental health.

CHAPTER 2

EMOTIONAL TENSION
AND YOUR EATING HABITS

Food swings can hinder or enhance your body's performance. Positive food swings brought on by healthy eating habits give you the horsepower to accomplish anything. But high stress levels make it hard to establish these wholesome eating habits, and so negative food swings follow. What do an arthritis-ridden housewife, a pilot with prostate cancer, and a burnt-out attorney have in common? They're all riding the roller coaster of dysfunctional food swings, caught in a cycle of high stress and improper diet.

Although stress is different things to different people, we can all identify it. Simply stated, stress is the stuff that makes you feel bad. When you're rushed, hassled, or pressured, challenges have crossed the line, transforming like Dr. Jekyll into a maniacal Mr. Hyde. Stress is a psychological burden that overloads your physical circuitry, setting up your body for one healing crisis after another. It's heavy. Traumatic life events, tough decisions, and adverse circumstances combine to make life very confusing.

Too many Americans subscribe to the Puritanical notion that stress makes you a stronger, sharper person. In fact, stress undermines your abilities, interferes with your performance, and zaps valuable energy. Stress is not the wind beneath your wings—it is the thundering storm that, in time, will tear off your wings. Prolonged stress is the leading cause of disease and premature aging in the United States.

To break the cycle of dysfunctional food swings, you need to know how to decrease the amount of stress in your daily life. Healthy eating habits can cut your stress levels down to size and reduce your fatigue.

EMOTIONAL DISTRESS DAMAGES THE BODY

Emotional stress can masquerade behind a variety of bad moods. Look for these warning signs: impatience, irritability, restlessness, hostility, defensiveness, frustration, forgetfulness, and anxiety. Others may accuse you of rudeness, insensitivity, or a short temper. In conversations, you may come across as distracted, disruptive, or overly aggressive. The sudden onset of irrational or hypercritical behavior is a sure tip-off that you're suffering from emotional stress.

We're all familiar with the general malaise caused by emotional stress: exhaustion, depression, insomnia. Inability to concentrate. Loss of self-confidence. Low self-esteem. Limited attention span. But prolonged unresolved stress turns into emotional distress that pushes the body to its breaking point. Defense mechanisms break down and immune systems weaken. Put more specifically, the strain can adversely affect your liver and adrenal glands, just as dysfunctional food swings can result in malnutrition.

From a practical viewpoint, emotional stress just consumes too much energy. Work habits change for the worse, absenteeism increases, financial prosperity declines. If at first you find it hard to get a handle on the health benefits of managing stress, then try thinking of the money!

EMT AND FINGERPRINT FOOD SWINGS

When you're stressed, Emotional Tension—I refer to it as EMT—accumulates. It's human nature to want to decompress the high level of EMT and thereby reduce tension, but we often rely on unhealthy methods. And there lies the origin of addictive eating habits and negative food swings.

Bottled-up feelings, repressed anger, and buried fears all bring your EMT to a boiling point. The high tension level triggers rotten moods. To cope, we search for comfort—a quick fix to relieve the stress. This need for relief is at the root of all addictions: food, alcohol, work, shopping, sex, gambling. We're often too preoccupied to pick up on the undercurrents, but recognizing the dynamics allows us to address the problem.

Our favorite foods are custom-designed to relieve EMT and effect an immediate mood change. They're available right now at a drive-through window or grocery store shelf near you. More than likely, they're already sitting in your cupboard or refrigerator, waiting for your next craving. They don't require any advance preparation—no time for second thoughts. Just pop the lid, rip the wrapper, and they're good to go. Your hand-to-mouth reflex can clock in at under 10 seconds.

Each person handles escalating EMT in a unique way, shaped by his or her individual mommy-daddy diet. Each person has his or her own finger-print food swings. The trick is to counter EMT by effectively resolving stressful issues, instead of falling back on familiar dysfunctional eating habits.

JENNIFER'S FIVE BUTTONS

Let's look at someone who exemplifies this situation. Jennifer had been trying to lose weight forever. In the past two years, she'd taken diet pills, water pills, and hormone shots. She'd tried two high-protein crash diets and had been to no fewer than four weight loss clinics. Nothing worked. The 5'9", 39-year-old schoolteacher came to my office complaining of stress, fatigue, and weight gain. "Dr. Meltzer," she said, "my glands aren't working anymore. I can't shake this fat loose." She weighed 175 pounds.

In spite of her self-diagnosis, there was nothing unusual about Jennifer's weight gain. She didn't have a glandular condition. She was overeating. After taking a thorough history and physical examination, I determined she had destructive eating habits and an inadequate exercise program to boot. Jennifer pleaded that she was too busy to exercise. The way she described her life, she was constantly climbing a wall of worry.

Aside from fighting the battle of the bulge, Jennifer found herself in the seventh year of a stressful marriage. Her eight-year-old daughter was driving her nuts. The only treadmill she found herself on was one of financial diffi-culties, marital discord, and work-related stress. She was contemplating throwing in the towel, quitting her job, and moving with her daughter back to her parents' home in Northern California.

Instead of helping her, Jennifer's body seemed to be working against her. She was struggling to hold on, but in the last year her mammogram revealed an abnormal lump, her PMS symptoms were worse than ever, and her fam-ily doctor had diagnosed her with sciatica (nerve pain in the back, hips, but-tocks, and thighs). At the time of our appointment, she was recovering from a second bout of bronchitis.

Jennifer's eating habits revealed the root of her health problems. She admitted she had a set routine, so it wasn't hard to evaluate. At the end of her work day, she'd pick up her daughter from school and head home. Once there, she'd thumb through the mail, put her things away, and change out of her work clothes. At this point, it would be about 4:00 in the afternoon. She'd then look around to make sure no one in the family was watching, and proceed to raid the refrigerator. She'd bring the food to her bedroom, and a tremendous sense of relief would wash over her as she indulged behind closed doors. For the climax of her daily feast, she'd down her favorite desserts from deep within the recesses of her closet. Indeed, Jennifer was a certified closet binger, burning herself out in a three-way tug-of-war between her husband, her daughter, and her job.

Despite the obviously destructive nature of her eating routine, Jennifer was reluctant to think of it as an emotional crutch. Moreover, she wasn't sure she was ready or willing to give up her daily ritual. At the same time, she said she was desperate for an answer to her predicament. I explained that her abusive eating patterns were prematurely aging her, and that, combined with the erratic emotional swings caused by her diet, they had put her on a colli-sion course with chronic illness—heart disease, diabetes, cancer.

I advised Jennifer to inventory her eating habits for five days using the survey in Chapter 1. She recorded the frequency with which she ate, the amount of food she consumed, her appetite at the time she ate, and her moods. I also emphasized that she pause to take account of her real feelings whenever she was compelled to overeat.

Just as 2 + 2 = 4, overeating equals high EMT. Always. Emotional depri-vation is the trigger that inevitably activates overeating. At the end of her self-survey, Jennifer and I concluded she had five broad buttons that set off her abusive food swings. She'd eat when she was:

1. Tired
2. Bored
3. Frustrated
4. Lonely
5. Depressed

Over the course of the next three months, Jennifer committed herself to conquering her negative food swings. She dug deep, and confronted her personal problems in all their complexity. It became clear to her that food was her best friend. She employed my techniques, particularly those geared toward healing emotional wounds and preventing negative food swings (outlined later, in Chapter 8). Within six months, she'd lost 40 pounds. That was three years ago. To my delight, Jennifer continues to maintain her weight loss.

WHO'S THE BOSS?

Jennifer experienced an "a-ha moment" when she realized that nutritious eating promotes not just physical but also emotional well-being. Healthy eating habits cause pleasurable food swings. They also protect the body from disease and decay, and increase energy. By recharging your cells, they give you an advantage in the workplace. You're calmer, you think more clearly, and you're in touch with your feelings. By extension, healthy food swings enhance your communication skills. All in all, they empower you to make the best use of your time.

Unhealthy eating habits, on the other hand, spread like weeds, insidiously undermining you. By degrees, these toxic behaviors infest the garden of your well-being. In the beginning, you may feel tired and anxious. Eventually, your illnesses will become more specific. Stubborn, undisciplined eating habits create arthritis of the mind as well as stiffness of the body. In fact, although it is rarely diagnosed as such, arthritis is often caused by improper diet. The hardening of the arteries can also be attributed to steady, self-abusive eating habits. But by the point that your condition is medically classifiable, you'll be so dependent on your destructive patterns that any stimuli—anxiety, fatigue, depression—will automatically provoke a binge. You'll be anaesthetized to your own emotions. By surrendering to stress, you're destined to become a casualty of dysfunctional food swings.

Like Jennifer, you're in charge of your own eating habits. You're the boss. You can accelerate the aging process and invite degenerative disease into your body, or you can take positive action and abolish your mommy-daddy diet before it destroys you.

THE RED LIGHT THEORY OF DYSFUNCTIONAL FOOD SWINGS

Even though disappointments and disturbances are a very real part of life, we are not usually prepared for these unhappy surprises, because few of us have been blessed with emotional mentors. Consequently, emotional ignorance becomes the norm. When you suppress or shut out bad feelings, you're vaguely aware that something's not right, but beyond that, you're clueless. You can't even define the problem, much less address it, and anyway, you're too distracted by the more immediate, tangible difficulties in your daily life-work issues, marriage issues, family issues. Your anxiety festers, your EMT escalates, and you rely more and more on your mommy-daddy diet for comfort, even though it seems to be helping less and less.

What happens if you run a red light at a busy intersection? Clearly, you put yourself at the very real risk of serious damage from oncoming cars. Stopping your car at a red light is a learned behavior. We're even tested on it before we're granted a driver's license. A red light is easy to spot, and its message is clear: Do not proceed until the light turns green. If you decided to *stop* stopping at red lights, you'd be deemed a menace to yourself and society, and your license would be revoked.

The human body does not come with traffic signals. Our nose does not light up at the first sign of stress. But EMT does alert us to rising stress. We just have to learn how to recognize our mind-body signals—the red lights of EMT—which, admittedly, are more subtle than crossing guards and traffic cops. If we ignore or overlook our internal stop signs, then, like a careless car driver, we're headed for a crash.

When you feel tense, stressed, rushed, or pressured, your EMT warning signal is flashing. As if you were driving a car, you need to slow down to a stop and think about your next course of action. Go through the red light, and you end up gorging late at night, or snacking as soon as you get home from work. In upcoming chapters, I'll discuss in detail how to respond to emotional red lights and resolve emotional conflicts.

Stress is here to stay, so the challenge is to keep EMT at a minimum. To resist the temptation of overeating, begin by taking full responsibility for your feelings. Calmly accept them. Don't stuff them into temporary silence. Experience your craving, but don't indulge it. It will pass. The honest admission that you are hooked on your unhealthy behavior, that you have chosen this behavior, and that you have the power to change this behavior, is an essential step toward overcoming dysfunctional food swings.

AVOID THE VACCINATION OF MEDIOCRITY

Imagine the anguish of waking up one day to realize you're old before your time. Your world is in pieces, life's passing you by. Why willingly subject yourself to such agony? You deserve better than McDonald's™ "break today," the burger, shake, and fries. You deserve a more energetic, fulfilling existence. So ask yourself what you're holding on to. Then let it go. Up to a point, poor health is reversible. Start now, and avoid the vaccination of mediocrity that immunizes the unexamined self. Will it be tough? Yes, occasionally. Sometimes you have to climb a couple of mountains and cross raging rivers to get to where you want to go. But aren't you bored with a body that runs on cruise control, when it has the potential for such higher performance?

Take a few minutes to inventory the relationship between stress and your eating habits by rating your Nutritional Discretionary Quotient (NDQ). Upon completion, total your score. Scores lower than 70 indicate that you have dysfunctional eating habits, and it's time for a change.

EMOTIONAL TENSION AND YOUR EATING HABITS

Test Your NDQ (Nutritional Discretionary Quotient)

_1 Always   _2 Usually   _3 Sometimes   _4 Rarely   _5 Never

1. I eat when I am emotionally upset. _____
2. I eat when I am depressed. _____
3. I eat when I am angry. _____
4. I eat when I am irritable. _____
5. I eat when I am tired. _____
6. I snack before going to bed. _____
7. I drink some alcoholic beverages prior to, during, or right after eating. _____
8. I lie to myself at least once a day about what I should be eating. _____
9. I am preoccupied with my dinner meal during my afternoon activities. _____
10. I find myself craving potato chips, pretzels, and party snacks at least once a week and sometimes once a day. _____
11. I find myself craving commercial ice cream at least once a week and sometimes once a day. _____
12. I find myself craving sweetened food and bakery goods. _____
13. I find myself craving meat at least once a week and sometimes once a day. _____
14. I find myself craving breads at least once a week and sometimes once a day. _____
15. I am accustomed to drinking beer or wine or other liquors with my meals even though I don't want to. _____
16. I have regular times each day that I eat dinner. _____
17. I chew each piece of food individually, one mouthful at a time, and avoid gulping. _____
18. I have a hearty appetite. _____
19. I chew each mouthful at least 10 and up to 25 times before swallowing. _____
20. I set aside worries and problems at mealtime. _____
21. I consistently undereat, or eat until I'm just full. _____

SCORE:

1. Never   _____
2. Rarely   _____
3. Sometimes   _____
4. Usually   _____
5. Always   _____
6. Total: _____

Making the connection between your EMT and your food swings enables you to map out a master plan, a counterattack that will help you to establish healthy food swings. In my Del Mar, California, clinic, we have a saying: "Pay Now or Pay Later." Make a conscious decision to alter your eating habits now, or deal with disease later.

CHAPTER 3

STRESSITION AND THE
THREE DEGREES OF BURNOUT

"**A**ntioxidant" **is one** of those official-sounding buzzwords that gets tossed around a lot these days, but what does it really mean? In general, oxidation describes the decay and deterioration of the body. Antioxidants, such as vitamin C, vitamin E, selenium, and zinc counter this aging process. They work to prevent cancer and other illnesses. Pro-oxidants, on the other hand, accelerate breakdown.

STRESS—A PRO-OXIDANT

Medical science has repeatedly proven that stress puts a heavy burden on the body. Stress generates toxins that oxidize, or cause chemical damage, to cells and tissues. There a three different types of stress:

1. Emotional

2. Environmental
3. Nutritional

Emotional stress can arise from professional pressures, marital problems, financial difficulties, and other personal conflicts. Anger, worry, fear, and fatigue can all create emotional toxins. Factors such as ultraviolet light, ionizing radiation, industrial pollutants, cigarette smoke, and contaminated water all fall under the category of environmental stress. Food additives and preservatives produce nutritional toxins.

The point being, stress of any sort results in toxins that chemically tax your systems.

OXIDATIVE STRESS DAMAGES YIUR TISSUES

Toxins, along with other stress-related, oxygen-based compounds such as peroxides, damage cells and tissues. Known collectively as "free radicals," they oxidize cell membranes as well as the DNA and mitochondria within each cell. Think of them as scavengers—these free radicals infest, then feed on, rotten tissue. The oxidative stress brought on by free radicals results in the biochemical degeneration of the body. **It's the human equivalent of rusting.**

STRESSITION IS THE OPPOSITE OF NUTRITION

We nourish and nurture our body with nutrition. When we eat properly and exercise body and mind, we attain a level of good health. On the other hand, when biochemical erosion results from a pile-up of oxidative stress, we suffer from what I call *stressition*. Stressition is the opposite of nutrition. It describes the way that we misfeed and generally damage our body in response to stress. Indications of stressition include fatigue, high blood pressure, allergies, indigestion, insomnia, headaches, backaches, and sexual dysfunction. Stressition causes an accumulation of oxidative stress which, in turn, causes cellular damage and chemical deterioration.

Oxidative stressition is the root of dis-ease. It inaugurates the transition from wellness to illness. By causing breakdowns in biophysical functions, it opens the door to serious sickness. As the cellular structure of vital organs is attacked, the damaged tissue begins to operate abnormally. Heart, kidney, and liver failure, hardening of the arteries, neurological problems, as well as all kinds of cancer can be attributed to prolonged stressition.

The following equation depicts the progress of oxidative stress:

Stress~>Toxins~>Free Radical Damage~>Oxidative Stress~> Abnormal Function~>Disease

Or, simplified:

Pro-oxidants~>Oxidative Stress~>Abnormal Function~>Disease

Different degrees of oxidative stressition take different tolls on the body. Mild oxidative stressition leads to premature burnout. Prolonged oxidative stressition accelerates the aging process. Advanced oxidative stressition triggers degenerative disease.

Emotional distress is the single most powerful cause of oxidative stress. A continuum of stressful events can lead to chronic emotional distress. Sadly, we've come to take such a condition as a given—a way of life. But the domino effect applies to emotional distress: In time, little bad habits become big bad habits, resulting in oxidative stress levels that corrode the nervous systems, glands, and vital organs.

After emotional distress, **nutritional distress is the second most common cause of oxidative stress.** A substantial percentage of daily stress can be traced to negative dietary choices. Refined foods laden with chemicals, or the acid toxins in red meat and poultry, to name two broad categories, have a damaging effect on your metabolism.

Emotional distress and nutritional distress are as interrelated as kissing cousins, because EMT—emotional tension—fuels nutritional tension. When you're emotionally stressed out, you're much more likely to indulge in abusive eating habits. EMT baits you. When you take the bait, and embark on a negative food swing, the subsequent nutritional distress invites disease. The following chart outlines how it all ties together.

THE WHEEL OF OXIDATIVE STRESS

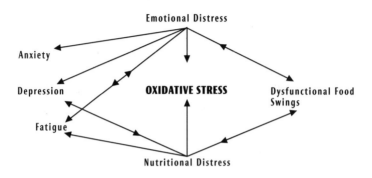

DEBBIE'S DILEMMA

Debbie had been feeling "under the weather" for the past five years. She was constantly afflicted with a sore throat, a bladder infection, and menstrual difficulties. Recently, she'd been experiencing numbness and tingling in her legs, as well as vision problems. At the ripe old age of 39, she found it tough to keep up with her two adolescent children. She let little things set her off and was quick to temper.

A local neurologist had diagnosed Debbie with early multiple sclerosis. He wanted to do more tests and prescribe various medications. Panicked, she came to me in search of an alternative approach to her predicament.

A complete physical examination revealed that Debbie was about 30 pounds overweight. She had a few scattered cysts in her breasts. Her vital signs were normal, but a neurological exam indicated that she had some mild difficulty with her gait and her equilibrium, along with some minor sensory deficits in the long nerves of her lower extremities. Experience has taught me that the early stages of oxidative stress and nutritional imbalance can often be misdiagnosed as multiple sclerosis, so I decided to get a more detailed, psycho-social history. This is what Debbie told me.

Debbie came from a small, conservative town about a half-hour drive from Green Bay, Wisconsin. Growing up, she'd had a good relationship with her mother, although they never discussed emotional issues. Her father was another story. Over the last ten years, Debbie had come to the realization that he did not know how to love her. He was aloof at family mealtimes, did not hug or kiss her, and did not express his affection in any way. Whenever she was lonely and confused, Debbie sought the advice of her best friend's father. By high school, she had learned to live with her family's "don't rock the boat" mentality.

In college, Debbie majored in English literature. A couple of years after graduating, she met Mack, who was then interning at a local hospital. They began dating, and when Mack got his surgical residency in Los Angeles, he asked Debbie to marry him and move to the West Coast. Although she was in the process of completing her master's degree in English, she figured she would finish her studies in California. In LA, she went to school three nights a week, and worked during the day at a dentist's office.

Mack had made it clear from the get-go that his career came first. When Debbie got pregnant, she stopped working, and had two children in as many years. Mack eventually finished his medical training, but the communication between the couple was strained. Preoccupied with his career and the financial responsibilities of raising two children, Mack became increasingly inaccessible. He was very similar to Debbie's father—same build, same voice, same opinions. He didn't share his feelings much.

Debbie desperately wanted her marriage to work, but the problems only escalated. After the birth of their second child, their sex life had fallen apart. One night, when their son was three and their daughter five, Mack came home from work and announced he wanted to marry the nurse in his office. Debbie was devastated. Her husband left her, and for the next nine years she worked her fingers to the bone, taking care of the kids and teaching English at the local high school. During that time, she'd had a few boyfriends, but found it difficult to trust men, and figured it was better for both her and her kids if she remained single. Mack supported the children financially, but he only saw them a couple of times a month.

The emotional stress in Debbie's life drove her to overeat. Everyday after work, she'd hit the road. That is, the rocky road. She stocked cartons of her favorite flavor ice cream in the freezer. After dinner and between meals, she craved cheese and crackers. As soon as the kids went to bed, she'd curl up with her favorite desserts and down them while watching TV or reading her romance novels.

I was sympathetic to Debbie's issues with men, and I understood how, between her family's tendency to ignore problems and her father's emotional remoteness, she ended up turning to food for comfort. But I explained to her that poor food choices could hurt and betray in their own, equally damaging, ways.

Prolonged emotional distress—compounded by the free radicals and toxins present in unnatural foods, refined carbohydrates, and fats—had left Debbie with a high level of oxidative stressition. Without wanting to frighten her further, I explained to Debbie that there was no time to hesitate. Her MS *would* worsen if she didn't take control of her life and commit to a complete nutritional and emotional detoxification.

Debbie confronted her demons and acknowledged that her dysfunctional food swings were an escape hatch that helped her avoid dealing with real issues. Over the next six months, she dedicated herself to high-performance nutrition. She stopped eating sweets, meats, soft drinks, dairy, caffeine, and white flour. She dedicated herself to the Rules for Healthy Food Swings that I'll outline in Chapter 6. She turned her health around. Four years later, all the symptoms of multiple sclerosis have disappeared, and the once-recurrent bladder and throat infections are long gone. Two years of therapy with a local psychologist helped her to resolve her trust issues. She's enjoying life with her two teenagers and is engaged to be married.

Different factors combine to make us who we are, and most of us carry childhood issues into our adult life, but there comes a time when we have to break the chain and claim responsibility. The level of your oxidative stressition is the sum total of your emotional and nutritional distress. And this is your own doing. Just as disciplined training is essential for athletic success and solid studying is necessary for academic achievement, so too are wholesome eating habits a requisite for good health. Healthy food swings prevent oxidative stressition.

In the next chapter, I'll identify the top ten foods that increase oxidative stress levels, but first let's review why oxidative stress is such a cause for concern:

- Oxidative stress disrupts the mind-body connection
- Oxidative stress devitalizes the immune system
- Oxidative stress precipitates target organ failure
- Oxidative stress leads to metabolic friction and metabolic burnout

OXIDATIVE STRESS DISRUPTS THE MIND-BODY CONNECTION

A balanced mind-body chemistry is essential for wellness. The ongoing, incredibly precise interactions of enzymes, hormones, neurotransmitters, and micronutrients determine this chemistry, affecting everything from physical performance to the ability to think. It's what makes you tick: Attitude, appetite, energy level, willpower, concentration, strength, stamina, behavior, and emotions all depend on the mind-body connection.

Your body is ingeniously equipped with a largely self-regulating pharmacy of enzymes, hormones, and neurological impulses. Thought, action, and emotion are all generated in the brain, home of the central nervous system. Then, through an elaborate network of nerve endings, impulses carry messages from mind to muscles in order to cause action. Glands—pituitary, thyroid, adrenal, gonadal, etc.—secrete hormones that affect your feelings, connecting them to ideas and behavior.

The state of your mind-body connection can be determined from the co-functioning of your nervous system and glandular metabolism, as governed by the neuro-chemical transmitters that carry messages. By depleting these neuro-chemical transmitters, oxidative stress disrupts the mind-body connection. The self-regulating pharmacy is sabotaged, throwing mind and body out of whack. All sorts of exhaustion occur: fatigue, lethargy, drowsiness, inertia. It becomes difficult to focus. Resolve weakens and willpower plummets.

The ironic thing is, most of us excuse our bad health habits because they temporarily relieve tension, but, by failing to nourish our blood and brain chemistries, these negative behaviors, and the oxidative stress they cause, worsen the situation.

OXIDATIVE STRESS DEVITALIZES THE IMMUNE SYSTEM

The immune system serves one crucial purpose: It protects you from illness. An efficient immune system fights off infections, viral insults, cancerous cells, and degenerative diseases such as multiple sclerosis. All great coaches know that a solid defense wins championships. Think of your immune system as your built-in linebackers. The key players? Your liver, spleen, lymph glands, and bloodstream.

Oxidative stress mounts an offensive against your immune system. It begins its attack by overloading your autonomic, or involuntary, nervous system. This nervous system, from your brain stem to your cranial nerves, intimately links to your immune system. By increasing tension in the involuntary nerve pathways, oxidative stress ultimately infiltrates the lines of defense, first causing liver stress and stress to the spleen. Then it goes on to debilitate lymphocytes and plasma. With a compromised immune system, too weak to fight off foreign invasion, you are more prone to the flu, bronchitis, soar throats, ear infections, and the like.

Moreover, the oxidative stress of repressed emotions drains the immune system. Buried fear, suppressed anger, and self-loathing all exacerbate stress levels. A weakened immune system factors into depression.

OXIDATIVE STRESS PRECIPITATES TARGET ORGAN FAILURE

"Psychosomatic" is just a more sophisticated way of referring to the mind-body connection: "psyche" refers to the mind, "somatic" to the body. Oxidative stress explains the psychosomatic origin of illness—the way we can literally worry ourselves sick.

Depending on such diverse factors as metabolism and genetic makeup, different people have different body targets that serve as the prime receptors of EMT. These targets are the organs most vulnerable to the displacement of emotional and nutritional distress. They're your body's weak spots, the areas where oxidative stress is stored and dietary toxins have the most severe impact. Some people experience migraine headaches, others stomach ulcers, and still others back pain. For example, Lisa and Scott, like so many married couples, share a similar diet. But when Lisa gets stressed out, she usually comes down with bronchitis, while Scott's body reacts to stress with acid indigestion. Sister and brother Careen and Ross are both attorneys in high-stress careers. Even though they were raised with the same diet, Careen is afflicted with arthritis, but Ross has high blood pressure. In order to effectively fight oxidative stress, it's essential to identify, and then take care of, your individual body targets.

Healthy food swings train your target organs to be strong. An energizing diet enables them to cope with the stression of everyday life. Impulsive eating binges, on the other hand, have the opposite effect. Choosing positive over negative food swings is one way to create psychosomatic (mind-body) balance.

OXIDATIVE STRESS LEADS TO METABOLIC FRICTION
AND METABOLIC BURNOUT

Your metabolism is your body chemistry. An efficient metabolism, one that makes the maximum use of nutrients and quickly disposes of any waste, is a key to sustained high-performance living. A gauge of your metabolic productivity can be gleaned by how often, and how much, you eat during a typical day. A healthy metabolism extracts a substantial amount of energy from significantly less food than we have been brainwashed into believing is a standard amount to consume.

Overeating is bad for your metabolism. Undereating is good. If you think of your body as a machine, undereating keeps the engine running and the gears clean. For example—and this flies in the face of what many so-called experts have been saying for years—**eating a big breakfast is one of the worst things you can do for your metabolism**—unless you've exercised extensively first, which most of us don't: Less than 10 percent of the U.S. actually works out before breakfast.

How long can you go without eating before your body craves food? The less often, and the less amount of food you have to eat to extract the necessary nutrients, the greater your metabolic efficiency.

Your metabolism is also the rate at which you burn fat, as indicated by your weight. Simply put, an efficient metabolism keeps hormones balanced, burns fat, and prevents weight gain. Conversely, an inefficient metabolism, one that is assaulted by oxidative stress, disrupts hormonal equilibrium, does not burn fat, and leads to weight gain. By impairing the function of key glands that regulate hormones, oxidative stress causes metabolic friction. For example, high levels of EMT adversely affect the thyroid and the pancreas. Thyroxin, produced by the thyroid, and insulin, secreted by the pancreas, both have a lot to do with whether you store or burn fat. Oxidative stress also impairs the hypothalamus, limbic system, and pineal glands. Overwhelmed by too much of the wrong type of fuel, the hormonal system loses its edge and begins to malfunction. The body's gears grind to a halt, and the decreased metabolism causes unwanted weight gain. Eventually, the engine breaks down.

In addition to overeating, other poor dietary habits cause metabolic malfunctions. Snacking on salty junk food, dairy-rich ice creams, caffeine-laced chocolate, and other high-sugar items negatively influences your nerves, hormones, and digestion by upsetting the delicate balance between proteins, carbohydrates, and fats.

Another psychosomatic way in which we derail our metabolism is through our anxiety. Often, the more nervous we are, the more irregular and abusive our eating habits. The metabolic friction caused by mental tension leads us to eat more in order to generate the same amount of energy. Over time, this pattern exhausts the metabolic machinery and it begins to malfunction, at which point we start to gain weight.

Metabolic friction—whether it's caused by overeating, poor nutrition, anxiety, or a combination of the three—is the reason why so many people who eat reasonably and exercise occasionally find it so easy to gain weight and so hard to lose it. Sporadic good habits can't fix a metabolism that's been severely damaged over time. Metabolic friction also leads to a smorgasbord of related weaknesses: functional reactive hypoglycemia, diabetes, liver dysfunction, pancreatic imbalances, adrenal deficiencies, hypothyroidism, anemia, and electrolyte disorders.

To summarize the effect of oxidative stress on metabolism:

- Your metabolism determines the rate at which you burn fat.
- Overeating impairs your metabolism by upsetting the balance of hormones that help to regulate how your body processes food.
- A poor diet impairs your metabolism by upsetting the balance between proteins, carbs, and fats.
- Anxiety impairs your metabolism by increasing the probability that you will engage in poor eating habits.

OXIDATIVE STRESS IS INEVITABLE, BUT . . .

As a doctor, I talk to different patients every day. After years of consultations, I've come to the conclusion that oxidative stress has reached epidemic proportions. It doesn't matter where you live, what your job is, whether you're single, dating, married, or divorced. Everyone everywhere is far too familiar with work pressures, financial strains, and relationship strife. People feel like their lives are spinning out of control. They're forever behind schedule. There's no time to relax. They rush from one moment to the next. They're tired, restless, frustrated, irritable. Their chaotic lifestyle leads to energy loss and weight gain.

Oxidative stress is a relatively recent phenomenon, and we're still wrestling with the reality that it has become a dominant, inescapable force. The technological revolution has left us on-line, in-line, maligned—everything but aligned. Each new advance designed to save time—cellular phones, e-mail, and so on—only seems to accelerate the pace. Oxidative stressition is spreading through our society like wildfire, burning out and breaking down every metabolism it comes in contact with. Burnout means you are out of touch with yourself and out of synch with your life. Stress, tension, fatigue, and depression are the cardinal symptoms of burnout. I've nicknamed this modern-day epidemic Tension-Fatigue Syndrome (TFS).

Don't try to deny it. Stress is getting to you. Admitting it is the first step toward addressing the problem. Why is the diagnosis of TFS so important? Because burnout, ignored or misdiagnosed, cannot possibly be properly treated. And without treatment, TFS snowballs. It progressively worsens to the point that it becomes chronic, or constant. The end result is degenerative disease and terminal illness.

When you are tired and tense for more than three weeks in a row, something is wrong. In fact, when you are tired and tense for more than three days in a row, it takes its toll. After six weeks these symptoms are a warning sign of impending chronic fatigue and subsequent chronic metabolic burnout. The snowball cycle of TFS can be simplified thus:

Oxidative Stress—>Tension-Fatigue Syndrome—> More Oxidative Stress—>Chronic Burnout—> Degenerative Illness (cancer, heart disease, stroke, liver failure, kidney failure, etc.)

To see how this sick cycle works, check out the graph below. I call it "Dr. Meltzer's Health Staircase." It descends to different levels, from wellness to disease. Optimum health ranks at 100, death at zero. Fifty marks the cut-off point between wellness and illness.

There are five fundamental categories of health:

1. Optimal Wellness
2. Partial Wellness
3. Average Health   ⎤ Burnout Zone
4. Poor Health   ⎦
5. Symptomatic Disease

These categories correspond to the five levels of immunological status as portrayed in the following graph:

DR. MELTZER'S HEALTH STAIRCASE

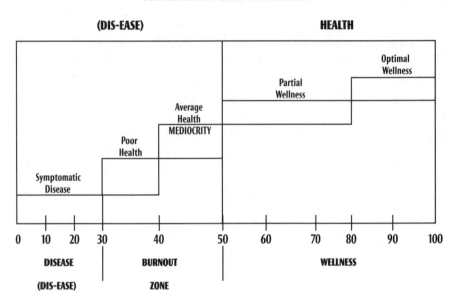

The human body is a tough, tenacious thing. It wants to live. Notice that it is not until you are operating at 30 percent of your maximum health that symptomatic disease and breakdown sets in. Your arteries can be 40, 50, even 70 percent clogged, and still you'll have no symptoms of heart disease. Your liver can be functioning at only 31 percent of its potential, and still all the tests on a blood panel will read normally. When you experience heart failure, stroke, cancer, arthritis, or the like—in other words, when you display the unmistakable symptoms of degenerative disease—your body has gone beyond the point of self-repair. The defense mechanisms of your immune system have broken down and decayed.

The top of the staircase, the level of **Optimal Wellness**, earns an "A" for excellence. This is the domain of high-performance living. Actually, 80, 90, and 100 can be ranked "A," "AA," and "AAA," respectively. As a member of the biophysical honor roll, you're physically fit, mentally clear, and emotionally balanced. Your energy level steadily sustains you for diverse, demanding days, and you need only a moderate amount of sleep at night. You transcend stress. You thrive.

Partial Wellness also can be registered at three levels: "B" for 50, "BB" for 60, and "BBB" for 70 out of a possible 100. Those of you on this step of the staircase look pretty good, and feel fine most of the time. You have a high energy level, although it could be higher. You're not operating at your maximum potential, but you're doing okay. Thanks to resourcefulness and resilience when faced with stress, you've managed to keep yourself from falling farther down. Your overall physical, mental, and emotional fitness help you stay in charge in your life. While you could be better balanced, in general you are not tired or irritable. But with a deeper commitment to your nutritional and emotional diets, you could be admitted to the A team. Consider upgrading your eating habits, simplifying your life, and devoting yourself with more passion to your physical self.

. . . BURNOUT IS REVERSIBLE

When you cross over to the left of center, you can see that there is a large section between Wellness and Disease. This is the Burnout Zone. It is crucial to distinguish between Burnout and Degenerative Disease. Metabolic burnout is reversible; degenerative disease is not. The three levels of burnout can be illustrated by the three lower steps on the staircase:

Average Health:	43–50	**first-degree burnout**
Poor Health:	34–43	**second-degree burnout**
Symptomatic Dis-ease:	31–34	**third-degree burnout**

As the above numbers indicate, once you hit the midway mark on the Stress Staircase, the rate of decline rapidly increases. Put another way, it's where the snowball really picks up speed.

Between the ages of 35 and 45, nearly 90 percent of Americans shift into first-degree burnout.

That's how prevalent oxidative stress is. And these days, those in their twenties and early thirties will tell you that oxidative stress comes knocking on their doors earlier and earlier. Unless first-degree burnout is recognized, treated, and reversed, by age 45, the second-degree stage of **Poor Health** sets in. By age 52 to 55, what started out as preventable, easy-to-fix, first-degree burnout can turn into terminal, third-degree burnout. The third degree is but a few heartbeats away from terminal **Symptomatic Dis-ease**.

Being at the bottom of the health staircase is like having one foot in the grave. Oxidative stression is on the brink of unleashing an irreversible degenerative disease. So take this opportunity to intervene. Teach yourself how to decrease oxidative stress and reverse burnout before it's too late.

JED FOUGHT FIRST-DEGREE BURNOUT

The cardinal symptom of first-degree burnout is fatigue. And I don't mean the normal physiological fatigue that occurs after a hard day's work. I'm talking about ever-present, bone-aching, headache-inducing exhaustion, the type that no amount of sleep seems to alter. Burnout appears gradually, and this dissipating energy level is the first way it makes itself known.

A number of factors may flick off the internal switch that keeps your energy flowing. The emotional distress inflicted by work, romantic, and parent-child relationships may be taking its toll. The nutritional distress of caffeine, sugar, alcohol or drug addiction may be depleting your reserves. To alter the course of first-degree fatigue, you have to take proactive steps, the same way Jed did.

At 38, Jed was struggling to keep up with his daily routine of work and child-rearing. He found himself fighting off mid-afternoon fatigue. Day in and day out, he felt more and more tired, and of late had lost the drive that used to fuel his professional performance. In the past two years, he had also gained 10 pounds, but it was tough to get to the gym. On the home front, he feared the passion had disappeared from his marriage.

Jed's primary physician could find nothing wrong with him. His cholesterol level was normal, and his blood tests showed no signs of disease. In fact, his doctor told him that his condition was to be expected. After all, he was nearing 40. But I could see that Jed was suffering from first-degree burnout—his declining energy and diminished enthusiasm gave it away. Other indications include weight gain and loss of libido. When you don't get a good night's sleep, you feel it the next day. You don't bounce back from the flu as quickly as you used to. In the early stages of burnout, you're still fighting the battle, but you're beginning to lose.

I prescribed the methods I'll describe throughout this book, and gave Jed specific, practical instructions on how to balance not just his diet, but his lifestyle. In addition to detoxifying his system with smart foods, he also increased his cardiovascular fitness and decreased his stress levels through regular meditation.

As Jed was happy to discover, the body's self-repair mechanisms can still be activated in the first-degree stage of burnout. With progressive levels of burnout, the corrective functions of the body cease to operate effectively and it takes longer to get over mental and physical setbacks. It's in the degenerative stage that corrective functions cease to operate.

THE SYMPTOMS OF BURNOUT

1°: Jed's story depicts the symptoms of first-degree burnout, a stage at which the body is still capable of curing itself. First-degree burnout is inconsistent. At times, you feel a sense of well-being, and you are not suffering from chronic mood swings, anxiety, lethargy, or depression. Mentally, you're mostly on the ball, able to concentrate, make decisions, and remember things. Physically, the signs of illness are transient: You do NOT have ongoing headaches, digestive difficulties, relentless allergies, recurrent flus, and chronic bronchitis. Maybe you've put on 10 to 20 pounds.

You still wake up each morning with the attitude that today, you're going to get things done. But your body just doesn't have enough energy anymore to deal with your unrealized dreams, unresolved feelings, and inescapable obligations.

2°: Oxidative stress is progressive. Left untreated, first-degree burnout quickly turns into intermediate, or second-degree, burnout. In this halfway house between fatigue and disease, the body experiences a more extensive exhaustion that is both physical and psychological. You carry on with your life, and rally to accomplish your chores with a reasonable amount of effort, but in second-degree burnout, your circuits are overloaded. It becomes more difficult to concentrate. Your irritability increases. Other symptoms include apathy, loss of ambition, sexual dysfunction, sleep disturbance, memory loss, indigestion, and irregular appetite.

The more extensive the burnout, the more significant the physiological warning signs. In the second-degree stage, blood pressure begins to rise. Headaches are common. You might have early signs of prostate dysfunction and the beginnings of arthritis. Allergies make breathing difficult. Cysts form. Insomnia takes hold. Relatively minor infections—sore throats and so on—are hard to shake. Dependence on alcohol, caffeine, sugar, and other substances contribute to the fatigue.

Second-degree burnout is often marked by a weight gain of 20 to 50 pounds.

With effort, the damage of second-degree burnout can be reversed. I have coached scores of people back from the brink of second-degree burnout into the wellness zone. The healing process requires a rigorous detoxification that treats both your negative food swings and their related emotional issues. But the payoff is well worth the work: You re-establish your momentum and regain your focus. You get well.

3°: One step above the bottom of the staircase, we hit third-degree burnout. And it hurts. It's not completely hopeless, and it's better than trying to turn back from the point of no return. Third-degree burnout can be coached back into the wellness zone, but it's an uphill battle. The majority of people who deteriorate to this extent lose ground and succumb to terminal illness. Disease takes over, and the body's self-regulating mechanisms, already weakened, struggle to engage in, literally, the fight of your life.

CHARTING BURNOUT

In essence, your level of burnout is determined by the extent, intensity, and duration of tension and fatigue. Using the chart below, identify your degree based on the column where you have the most marks.

	1°	2°	3°
Fatigue	Tiredness	Lethargy	Exhaustion
Stress Level	High	Very High	Overwhelming
Energy Level	Low	Very Low	Extremely Low
Weight Gain	Mild (10–20 lb)	Moderate(20–50 lb)	Severe (50+ lb)
Depression	No	Yes	Advanced
Anxiety	Sometimes	Usually	Always
Mood Swings	Rare	Occasional	Frequent
Memory Loss	Rare	Occasional	Frequent
Insomnia	Rare	Occasional	Frequent
Sexual Dysfunction	Sometimes	Usually	Always
Attitude	Neutral	Negative	Very Negative
Signs and Symptoms of Illness (e.g., high blood pressure, arthritis)			
	Mild	Moderate	Severe
BURNOUT LEVEL	MILD	MODERATE	SEVERE

OXIDATIVE STRESS CAUSES PTA BURNOUT

No, PTA Burnout doesn't refer to what happens when you volunteer for too many of your kid's school and extracurricular activities. "PTA" is an abbreviation for your **P**ituitary-**T**hyroid-**A**drenal axis. Oxidative stress puts pressure on your brain—specifically the hypothalamus and limbic system, two areas where emotions are generated. The tension is then transferred to your pituitary, the master endocrine gland at the base of the brain. The pituitary regulates your adrenals and thyroid, the two glands that, in turn, regulate your metabolism. This Pituitary-Thyroid-Adrenal axis, along with your liver and kidneys, determines your daily energy level. So it stands to reason that a well-managed stress level puts less strain on your brain and leaves you with lots more energy.

Relaxation revitalizes your PTA axis. Oxidative stress alarms it. You're probably already familiar with the PTA response to crisis: We commonly call it the "fight or flight" mechanism. When, for example, you fear an oncoming car, your pituitary secretes ACTH (Adreno-Cortico-Trophic Hormone), a messenger hormone that tells the adrenal glands to release adrenaline and other stress-related hormones. Adrenaline stimulates your body, so that you sprint out of the way before the car gets too close. By the same token, when you are under constant emotional stress, your pituitary secretes TSH

(Thyroid-Stimulating Hormone), another messenger, which tells the thyroid gland to release thyroxin. Thyroxin keeps you mentally alert, so that you are able to deal with the stress at hand. Problem is, when you are under constant stress, your thyroid—and, by extension, your PTA axis—gets overactivated. Excess hormone production takes place in the adrenal and thyroid glands, until your stress levels exhaust their hormonal reserves. The resulting imbalance causes fatigue. Standard medical blood tests may be normal, because labs look for outright deficiencies, not more subtle imbalances. Granted, the adrenal and thyroid glands have not gone into failure. Yet. But consider your increasing fatigue as a serious warning sign.

And that's the energy-depleting cycle of stressition: Oxidative Stress drains the nerves, overstimulates the glands, and imbalances the hormones. As your body's biochemistry readjusts to the stress assault, it depletes the reserves of stress-related hormones intended to fight off legitimate life-threatening illness. Chronic fatigue sets in. One way to avoid this all-too-common syndrome is to identify those foods that increase stress levels. That's what we do next.

CHAPTER 4

KEEPING YOUR SYSTEM RUNNING CLEAN:
HOW TO AVOID THE TOP TEN ANTI-NUTRIENT FOODS

Most of us *think* we know how to eat right, even if we don't know the effect each food has on our body. We've seen the FDA-approved food pyramid on the back of cereal boxes, the one that suggests ten servings of breads, grains, and pasta per day. But this standardized American diet is actually dominated by anti-nutrients.

All foods contain a range of chemical components that include nutrients. Nutrients are the life-giving elements in food that nourish you. There are three categoties of **nutrients: nutrients, phytonutrients,** and **co-nutrients. Essential nutrients**, such as vitamins, minerals, and amino acids (the building blocks of protein) contribute to cell structure and physiological functioning. **Phytonutrients**, such as flavonoids and carotenes, protect the body from cancer and the damaging effects of free radicals. **Co-nutrients**, such as enzymes and fiber, also provide substantial health benefits. Nutrients nurture and nourish the body. **Anti-nutrients** do exactly the opposite. They deplete and weaken. The only thing they increase is your oxidative stress level.

Anti-nutrient foods are either lacking in nutrients to begin with or have been stripped of positive components in the refining process. White bread, for example, loses much of its vitamin and fiber content. When your body encounters anti-nutrients, in order to metabolize and eliminate them, it uses up its own reserve of vital nutrients. **By thwarting your body's efficient utilization of nutrients, anti-nutrients interfere with your metabolism.** By extension, they devitalize the immune system, accelerate the aging process, and put you at risk for illness.

Anti-nutrients undo mind-body balance.

ANTI-NUTRIENTS PROVOKE LIVER STRESS AND KIDNEY STRESS

Think of the liver's awesome job. It keeps the body clean. It is responsible for metabolizing everything you consume, including fatty foods, artificial flavorings, high-cholesterol meats, and over-acidic chicken, shellfish, junk foods, and soft drinks. (Specifically, the liver utilizes the cytochrome P450 enzyme system to reduce or hydrolyze the toxic impact of anti-nutrients.) By increasing the toxic load on your liver, anti-nutrients stress out this vital organ.

You could say that the liver has a brain. It knows what is good for it, and what is bad. It battles anti-nutritional bad guys with detoxification, its ingenious auto-regulatory process. But, like Superman to kryptonite, the liver is not invulnerable. Number one, the organ is overworked, and its chronic stress load decreases its efficiency. Number two, in the process of countering the assault of anti-nutrients, free radicals are generated, thereby further increasing the liver's stress level.

To inactivate the toxins that work their way into the body, the liver needs a steady supply of specific valuable nutrients. This nutritional arsenal includes vitamins B_1, B_2, B_3, and B_6, folic acid, magnesium, selenium, phosphatidylcholine (also known as lecithin), and zinc. The more anti-nutrients you have in your body, the more your liver must rely on its arsenal to detoxify them; and the more the liver relies on the arsenal, the less chance there is for the valuable nutrients to serve their proper metabolic purpose.

For their part, the kidneys maintain the alkaline-acid balance of bodily fluids. Plasma, spinal and joint fluids, and cells all function best in an alkaline medium. But certain anti-nutrients over-acidify the bloodstream and stress the kidneys. By doing so, they interfere with the kidneys' balancing act.

Anti-nutrients are internal garbage. They produce toxins and free radicals. They cause structural damage to cells. They promote organ dysfunction. They put you at risk for third-degree burnout.

In fact, I cannot think of a single nice thing to say about them.

CLEANSE YOUR BODY OF ANTI-NUTRIENTS

Eliminating anti-nutrient foods from your diet goes a long way toward alleviating the oxidative stress of modern-day living. If we think back to the body-engine metaphor, it's only logical that we should strive to keep our engine parts—blood, liver, kidneys, and spleen—clear of the debris, grease, and grime that anti-nutrients can deposit. Vital organs are popular lodging spots for these devitalizing devils, which can even penetrate bones and muscles. But I'm going to tell you how to give your liver and kidneys a break.

THE TOP TEN ANTI-NUTRIENTS THAT INCREASE OXIDATIVE STRESS LEVELS

1. WHITE REFINED SUGAR
2. WHITE REFINED CARBOHYDRATES AND WHITE FLOUR
3. PROCESSED AND SATURATED FATS
4. JUNK FOODS
5. DAIRY PRODUCTS AND EGGS
6. MEAT PROTEINS
7. SOFT DRINKS
8. CAFFEINE
9. ALCOHOL
10. SALT

Just Say No to Anti-Nutrients

I bet you see some of your favorite things on that Top Ten list. Who doesn't? But look at it this way: Anti-nutrients trigger oxidative stress. They lead to fatigue, anxiety, depression, mental dullness, and emotional shutdown—all symptoms of burnout. They result in hazardous food swings, and invite meta-bolic imbalance by overworking the liver, kidneys, pancreas, and adrenal glands.

Again, I cannot think of a single nice thing to say about them.

It's difficult to let go of American dietary staples such as milk, hamburg-ers, ice cream, coffee, and beer, and substitute them with healthy alterna-tives such as rice milk, garden burgers, fruit salads, and herbal teas. But I don't expect you take my word at face value. Find your favorite items on the Top Ten list, then check out what they're really doing to your body:

1. White Refined Sugar:

White refined sugar, or **sucrose**, drains your liver, imbalances your adre-nal glands, overtaxes your nerves, and depletes your B vitamins. It con-tributes to allergies, arthritis, premenstrual syndrome, and abnormal hor-monal fluctuations in both women and men. It is the root cause of func-tional hypoglycemia (low blood sugar). It accelerates the onset of adult dia-betes (high blood sugar). Perhaps most commonly, by setting up the body's energy level to hit a false peak and then crash back down, it causes chronic fatigue and an unstable metabolism.

Sugary sweets are associated with pleasure. Think of all the affectionate terminology we attach to the mere idea of sugar, from sweetheart to sweet tooth. Sweets have become hopelessly linked to happiness, and they often make up a large part of most mommy-daddy diets. Are all sugars the same? Are certain candies and cookies better for you than others? Let's trace the trajectory of refined white sugar in the body's systems.

Sweet and Low: the Story of the Sugar Blues

After you eat refined white sugar, it is rapidly absorbed right into the blood-stream. Your blood sugar is immediately raised, and the energy rush gives you a temporary high. You feel good. But to regulate this blood sugar rush, your pancreas quickly secretes an intense amount of insulin. The insulin lowers your blood sugar but, because it was forced to respond so quickly and intense-ly, it overcompensates, and you come crashing down. That's the sugar cycle.

The sugar cycle is one of the most common, and aggravating, food swings. In fact, it exemplifies the notion of a negative food swing, because it literally sends your metabolism up and down, high and low, much too fast. The rapid decline in blood sugar level leads to the sugar blues: fatigue, anxiety, and irritability follow the brief burst of energy. And the typical response is to eat *more* sugar, which only repeats the cycle.

White refined sugar is not natural. It is man-made. By the way, the same way that sucrose pollutes the body, so too does the manufacturing of sucrose pollute the environment. Sugar cane, for example, is considered a mineral-hungry plant that depletes soil. Common sugar-cane farming techniques employ substantial amounts of pesticides and fertilizers.

When whole sugar cane is converted into refined white sugar, it is stripped of essential minerals and vitamins. Once in your system, refined white sugar steals back its missing nutrients from your liver. Because it has no other way of metabolizing and digesting sucrose, the liver has to comply. So white refined sugar not only deprives your body of the nutrients that can be found in natural sugars, but also depletes the few key nutrients your body has in storage. Over time, the consumption of refined-sugar sweets leads to liver stress and nutritional deficiencies.

In spite of its candyland, lollipop image, white refined sugar is not pretty. Eating sucrose-laden products, even just a couple of times a week, leads to liver, adrenal, and pancreatic stress, which, in turn, can cause either functional hypoglycemia or acquired adult diabetes. White refined sugar is also a culprit in everything from common colds and flu, bronchitis, sinus infections, and digestive difficulties to breast cancer, Alzheimer's disease, and candida. By weakening the immune system, it increases the risk of degenerative illnesses and infections. In addition to imbalancing the pancreas and liver, it also attacks the central nervous system. It kills brain cells. **Avoid this vicious anti-nutrient in all its guises:** candies, chocolates, cake, ice cream, donuts, pastries, jams and jellies, and artificial sweeteners such as mannitol, saccharin, Equal™, and Nutrasweet™. And watch out for the refined white sugar present in brown sugar, turbinado sugar, and high-fructose corn syrup.

2. Refined White Carbohydrates and White Flour:

Complex carbohydrates, such as those found in whole grain breads, cereals, and pastas, contain a cornucopia of minerals, vitamins, and enzymes. But when whole grains are refined, vital nutrients are extracted. White bread, white rice and noodles, white flour, commercial breakfast cereals, soda crackers, and flour tortillas have all been "blanched" of their nutritional value.

Put simply, they're naked.

In a process similar to the one described above for refined white sugar, refined white carbohydrates exhaust the body's supply of key B vitamins and essential minerals such as calcium, magnesium, and zinc. They impair the liver's detoxifying functions. Furthermore, they are much lower in fiber than their whole grain equivalents. White rice, which many Americans consider to be a healthy food choice, actually has zero nutrients and zero fiber.

Processed carbohydrates pollute the body. They are not a "clean" food— they leave behind a pasty mucus that coats the respiratory, nervous, lymphatic, and digestive systems. This thick sludge causes disorders like constipation, spastic colon, irritable bowel syndrome, and diverticulitis. White flour, as found in white bread, macaroni, and packaged breakfast cereals, can also be mucus-forming. The resulting clogged lymphatic system increases susceptibility to colds, the flu, and bronchial and sinus infections. And white flour contains ailoxan, a diabetes-promoting substance. Not to mention that excess consumption of all those carbs, from white pasta to white crackers with cheese, damages your body's ability to burn fat and leads to weight gain.

A simple rule: Stay away from white foods.

3. Processed and Saturated Fats:

It's no secret that a high fat diet is hazardous to your health. High fat levels impede circulation and cause such major-league diseases as hardening of the arteries, blood clots, diabetes, stroke, and heart attack. High fat levels also increase the risk of breast, uterine, and gall bladder cancer. A high fat diet plays a causative role in the formation of gallstones, and negatively alters the chemical composition of bile, which is essential to the liver's detoxifying process. On a more basic level, before the body reaches any of the aforementioned crisis points, a high fat diet, of course, results in obesity.

But not all fats are off-limits. To their credit, fats—made up of building blocks known as fatty acids—provide a concentrated source of energy. The four general categories of fats are:

Saturated Fats: Bad. Saturated fats, typically of animal origin, are high in cholesterol and have been linked to the onset of cancer, particularly breast cancer. Examples of saturated fats include: bacon, ground beef, butter, cream cheese, ice cream, coconut oil, palm oil, hydrogenated oils, lard, sausage, and whole milk.

Monounsaturated Fats: Good. Monounsaturated fats have been shown to lower blood cholesterol levels. They are predominantly from the plant kingdom, and tend to clean out, rather than clog, arteries. Almonds, avocados, canola oil, olive oil, and peanuts are high in monounsaturated fats.

Polyunsaturated Fats: Good AND Bad. Polyunsaturated fats are nicknamed "the in-between fats" because they have both positive and negative properties. The problem with polyunsaturated fats is, when they are exposed to heat or sunlight, they generate free radicals. Safflower, sunflower, and corn oils, followed by peanut oil, are high in polyunsaturated fats.

Trans-fatty Acids: Bad. Trans-fatty acids are man-made, and are considered by some in the medical profession to be even more harmful than saturated fats. They are thought to play an active role in the hardening of arteries, and are also considered a risk factor for heart disease. They raise bad low-density lipoprotein (LDL) cholesterol and lower beneficial high-density lipoprotein (HDL) cholesterol. In addition to cardiovascular disorders, trans-fatty acids have also been linked to cancer, diabetes, and infertility.

Labels do not list trans-fatty acids, but they are present in: all refined oils; margarine, hydrogenated peanut butter, and other spreads; commercially baked cookies and cakes; and fried foods. When polyunsaturated oils such as safflower, sunflower, and corn oil are heated, trans-fatty acids are produced. It's best to avoid all hydrogenated oils, but if you're dead set on using margarine, buy one that is not hydrogenated.

A Sticky Situation: Canola or Olive Oil?

Because of its low levels of saturated fat and its relatively high poly- and monounsaturated fat content, canola oil is an acceptable choice—but olive oil is better. Olive oil offers the greatest health benefits: It is high in monounsaturated fats and it does not break down into trans-fatty acids when heated. Fresh virgin olive oils are light and easy to digest. Their delicate aroma and subtle flavor enhance most foods. Olive oil also contains valuable nutrients.

In a nutshell:

- Use olive oil
- Avoid tropical oils
- Eliminate hydrogenated oils
- Trash trans-fatty acids

Be On Guard For Bad Fats

Unfortunately, today's technology—solvent extraction, degumming, bleaching, deodorizing, and mechanical pressing—ends up excising the nutritional value from most commercial cooking oils. These oils are also subjected to pressure and high temperatures, sometimes in the presence of aluminum, which has been shown to increase the risk of Alzheimer's. Cheap, spreadable margarines, shortenings, and partially hydrogenated vegetable oils are all produced through this process.

Fats found in meat, lard, and dairy are high in cholesterol. Be suspicious of labels that announce "zero cholesterol," because the products probably contain trans-fatty acids such as those found in margarine, egg substitutes, or vegetable shortening. It's wise to eliminate these synthetic fats altogether.

4. Junk Foods:

Most Americans are on a first-name basis with their neighborhood fast-food emporium. The statistics are overwhelming: The average American consumes more than 125 pounds of sugar a year, 250 pounds of meat, 125 pounds of fat, and nearly 300 cans of soda. Although the rest of the world regards our eating habits with disgust and dismay, their own cultures are increasingly susceptible to them. How ironic is it that McDonald's™ was the main sponsor of the 2000 Olympics? It's embarrassing to be credited with ruining the world's diet and creating a generation of obese children, especially when the alternative is so simple.

Junk foods, loaded with chemicals, additives, pesticides, and preservatives, are mega-anti-nutrients. The name says it all: They're garbage, detritus, waste. Junk foods pile on the empty calories—all you gain from them is weight. And even though we're more educated about food than ever before, our dependence on junk only seems to increase. Superstar athletes send a mixed message by endorsing fast-food chains, and televised sporting events are interspersed with commercials for southern fried chicken and bacon double cheeseburgers. Misleading information dominates the media. Thanks to incessant advertising, the general public has been persuaded that fast food gives the greatest satisfaction. On top of that, stress levels have reached such high proportions that people choose the convenience and immediacy of fast food over the long-term benefits of more nutritional eating—they'd rather wolf down their meal and get back to work than slow down and savor healthier meals. Finally, many of us have become almost inextricably emotionally attached to our beloved junk food. We can't bear the thought of parting ways.

Because many of us have been brought up on junk, we don't even like the taste of natural food. It's important to allow yourself time to work through this dilemma when first confronting your unhealthy diet. The body develops habits over the course of many years of abuse. As with any other addiction, it's tough to quit cold turkey or change overnight. Taste buds become accustomed to the stimulants, such as sugar, salt, and additives, found in junk food. At first, fresh carrot or watermelon juice may be unappetizing. But eating well for 21 days—that's only three weeks—will alter your body's disposition, and it will begin to crave fruits, vegetables, and whole grains.

There's no question: junk foods accelerate oxidative stress. They upset the balance of the liver and the spleen by making them work in overdrive to detoxify all the chemicals. It takes some determination to abandon all the packaged products that line the shelves of supermarkets and can even be picked up without ever getting out of your car, but the difference in your health will be dramatic.

5. Dairy Products and Eggs:

Plainly put, dairy products are high-fat foods that increase liver stress. The intake of eggs and dairy items—pasteurized milk, hard cheese, ice cream, yogurt, and the like—strongly correlates to the incidence of cardiac arrest, diabetes, and cancer. Dairy products have been linked to such seemingly diverse disease states as cataracts, colitis, multiple sclerosis, and arthritis. Milk proteins have just as many anti-nutrients as meat proteins, and produce autoantibodies (antibodies that attack the tissues that produce them) associated with lupus, scleroderma, and other connective-tissue and autoimmune disorders.

By overstimulating the upper respiratory passages, dairy products provoke the excess secretion of mucus. The resulting layer of bio-slime creates all sorts of problems. It prevents the body from fighting off viruses, and leads to ear infections, sinus infections, bronchitis, tonsillitis, sore throats, and common colds. Mucus in the intestinal tract compromises digestive functions, causing such disorders as lactose intolerance and diarrhea. Undiagnosed food allergies responsible for everything from asthma to fatigue can be traced to dairy products.

After studies confirmed that dairy cows treated with bovine growth hormone (BGH) had significantly shorter life spans than those that were not, the steroid came under scrutiny. As you wean yourself off dairy items, check the labels to confirm that the manufacturer does not use BGH.

Got Milk?

In recent years, milk has been heavily promoted, particularly to teenagers and menopausal women, as an essential provider of calcium for strong bones. The dairy industry wants you to believe that bone loss is due to the diminished intake of dietary calcium, and they've lined up the sexiest celebrities to make their pitch. **Don't buy the dairy myth that milk prevents osteoporosis.** It has been scientifically proven that the excess consumption of dairy and meat increases the body's acid content. In other words, *dairy and meat cause calcium to be withdrawn from bone structures.* So don't believe the hype. It's true that some 25 percent of women age 65 or older suffer from severe bone mineral losses, and that the number of deaths due to osteoporosis equals those caused by breast cancer. But not only do dairy products *not* address the problems behind this epidemic, they exacerbate them.

Egg Consumption = Phlegm Production

Eggs are an even more dominant food allergen than dairy proteins. In my practice as a family physician, I can't begin to count the thousands of kids I have treated that had been prescribed unnecessary antibiotic therapy when, in fact, they were simply allergic to eggs. **Egg white, or albumin protein, is extremely allergenic,** especially in children. More kids visit the pediatrician each year for ear infections and sore throats caused by albumin allergies. Entire epidemics of colds and flu are misdiagnosed.

And by now everybody ought to know that **egg yolks are loaded with cholesterol**.

Eggs also have the dubious honor of being **the most mucus-forming food**. They cause sinus and lymph congestion as well as all the other phlegm-related problems described above for dairy products. Steer your family away from them! If you have young children, provide them with the proteins they need for healthy growth by serving alternatives such as rice milk, almond-sesame milk, or soy milk. For even greater nutritional value, add brewer's yeast. Scrambled tofu makes an excellent substitute for scrambled eggs, and soy products counter the over-proteinization caused by too much dairy. By eliminating eggs and dairy from your household's diet, you can dramatically reduce your risk of colds and flu—upper respiratory infections that drain your body of energy.

6. Meat Proteins:

Americans can attribute practically all of their consumption of saturated fats to meat proteins. The accumulation of such fats leads to *atherosclerosis*—more commonly known as hardening of the arteries. Blocked arteries can be credited for a number of life-threatening conditions, including heart arrhythmia, coronary disease and cardiac arrest, hypertension, stroke, memory loss, and dementia. As I mentioned earlier, when describing the detriments of dairy products, animal proteins deposit a toxic overload of acid that leaches calcium from the bones and predisposes the body to osteoporosis, arthritis, and rheumatism.

Considered carcinogenic, meat proteins are suspected to increase the risk of colon, pancreatic, breast, and prostate cancer. In addition to their high saturated fat content, they are spiked with artificial preservatives and other chemicals that stimulate overeating, and they contain absolutely no fiber.

Because the food industry is always changing its tune, most people today have been convinced to cut back on their consumption of red meat and pork in favor of leaner chicken and fish. But keep in mind that fish—particularly shellfish—also contain cholesterol and saturated fat. Most fish have a high amount of mercury, a toxic heavy-metal anti-nutrient that damages nerve, liver, and brain tissues. But my greatest concern with fish—and again, particularly shellfish—is the risk of contamination. Industrial and agricultural chemicals in our waterways are absorbed by fish through their skin into the bloodstream, and end up in the muscles. As large fish eat smaller fish, the contamination becomes more concentrated. Salmon, whitefish, and swordfish often contain high levels of PCB and other pesticides. Chicken protein is no prizewinner, either. Chicken meat causes hormonal imbalances in both genders, and may increase the risk of breast or prostate cancer. For more information on the damaging effects of animal proteins, read John Robbins' *Diet for a New America*.

From a more holistic, mind-body point of view, the most compelling reason not to eat animal proteins has to do with the adverse impact meat has on your soul. Yoga, a 5,000-year-old discipline, teaches that meat proteins suffocate and retard your spiritual development. Of course, each individual needs to come to terms with such issues in his or her own time. **To start, honestly examine how you feel before, during, and after you eat meat protein.** In spite of the current craze for high-protein diets, common sense alone should convince us that fatty, chemically enhanced, non-fibrous, acid-depositing meats are blatantly anti-nutritious.

7. Soft Drinks:

Caffeinated sodas are a cultural phenomenon. Coca-Cola™, Pepsi™, and other brands outsell fruit and vegetable juices by an alarming margin. But soft drinks are far from soft. High in phosphorous and phosphoric acid, they infiltrate bodily fluids and corrode stomach linings, upset the alkaline-acid balance of the kidneys, and eat away at your liver like Hannibal Lecter. Soft drinks also contain hidden caffeine, refined sugar, and artificial chemicals.

8. Caffeine:

With the custom-coffee trend showing no sign of slowing down, caffeine has become a billion-dollar industry, ranking right up there with sodas and sweets. In some ways, coffee has replaced alcohol and drugs: People consider it a legal, safe way to give themselves a jump start, especially in the morning, and they're comforted by the new café culture. Espresso bars are places to hang out, read, socialize, and soak up the rich aroma of freshly brewed exotic beans. The average American consumes at least two cups of coffee, or about 200 milligrams of caffeine, daily.

But caffeine overstimulates the nerves and glands. It drains the adrenal system, damages the thyroid, and can trigger heart arrhythmias. In female *and male* menopause, caffeine plays a role: Breast cysts and lumps are common in women, while men suffer from caffeine-induced prostate problems.

Chronic caffeine consumption causes a dysfunctional food swing similar to the sugar cycle: a peak in nervous energy, followed by a drastic drop into depression and irritability. Symptoms include headaches, heart palpitations, and insomnia. Anxiety-prone individuals and those under stress are particularly sensitive to the effects of caffeine. As with any other addiction, though, caffeine is tough to kick, because the symptoms of withdrawal can be painful, and depression and anxiety initially worsen.

In fact, coffee with milk and sugar presents a triple threat to your health: caffeine, dairy, and sucrose. So wake up and smell the java—just don't drink it.

9. Alcohol:

A depressant, alcohol dulls the brain and nervous system. It also wreaks havoc with the liver, overstimulates the adrenal glands, and disrupts sleep patterns. There are escalating degrees of alcohol consumption, from alcohol use, to alcohol abuse, to alcohol dependency and full-blown alcoholism. Alcohol-dependent individuals often suffer from depression, and medical experts concur that this is at least partially due to the fact that substantial alcohol intake exhausts levels of the essential amino acid tryptophane. Normally, tryptophane converts to serotonin, an important neurotransmitter and natural tranquilizer responsible for elevating and stabilizing mood. But alcohol interferes with the serotonin metabolism. When tryptophane levels are lowered due to alcohol consumption, then serotonin levels are also lowered, leading to depression.

Because alcohol damages intestinal microflora, it causes the malabsorption of fats, carbohydrates, and proteins. Alcohol also lowers blood sugar, thereby increasing cravings for sweets. A classic anti-nutrient, it depletes vitamins A, B, and C, folic acid, magnesium, and zinc. Heavy drinkers who happen to be weight-conscious often take shortcuts in their diets, because alcohol contributes a significant amount of empty calories. As a result, they usually exhibit deficiencies in vitamin E, selenium, and trace minerals. Alcohol elevates free radical levels, increasing oxidative stress. Learn to limit liquor intake to special occasions in order to avoid abusing this legal drug.

10. Salt:

The salt shaker can be a deadly weapon. With a proper potassium-to-sodium ratio, the body can maintain an efficient metabolism and immune system, but a high intake of salt—sodium chloride—drives out potassium. The imbalance upsets plasma and joint and spinal fluids. Fruits and vegetables, as part of a cleansing raw-food diet, can provide a potassium-to-sodium ratio of 100 to one. But most people have more salt in their diet than potassium, and a potassium-to-sodium ratio of six to one is considered optimal. The majority of Americans have a ratio of *salt to potassium* of two to one.

Too much salt at the expense of potassium results in high blood pressure. It also leads to edema and water retention, especially in women during the last half of their menstrual cycle. Excessive salt intake causes kidney stress, once again deregulating the body's natural alkaline-to-acid balance. Salt also disturbs digestion, and has been linked to stomach cancer.

Salt cravings, typified by potato chip binges and a lust for nuts, make up some of the most common food swings. Even though the human body can get the necessary amount of salt naturally, by eating fruits, vegetables, whole grains, and beans, 50 percent to as high as 80 percent of sodium in the average American diet comes from adding it to food while cooking.

Reduce foods that fall into any of these Top Ten categories, and you'll instantly reduce your oxidative stress levels. For my two formulas to further eliminate stress and overcome burnout, read on.

CHAPTER 5

CONQUERING STRESS:
WHAT YOU *REALLY* NEED TO KNOW

Stress is a sad fact of life, but that doesn't mean you have to lie down like a dog and take it. For your body's sake, fight back! If you don't do something about stress, it most certainly will do something to you.

The clock is ticking.

There's no time to waste.

Those who conquer their stress levels control their life. Their mind-body balance enables them to prosper at home, at play, and at work. Imagine how wonderful each day would be if you had more energy, more enthusiasm, more passion. Imagine how much better you'd feel about yourself if you actually *liked* what you saw when you looked in the mirror. Body confidence extends to every area of your life, from your ability to get along with coworkers to your sex appeal. Oxidative stress, on the other hand, can be compared to one big, wet blanket, suffocating your personality, extinguishing your spirit, and accelerating your rate of aging. Don't let stress destroy the natural rhythm of life: Follow my lead, and let me show you how to get in touch with yourself.

PRO-CHOICE

Hard as it may be to believe, good health is yours for the taking. It's not a matter of chance, a question of luck: It's your choice. Choose life now! Right now. Tomorrow never comes, and waiting—until next week, or after the holidays, or after you turn 50, or after your next promotion, or after any of the other little milestones we use to postpone dealing with our daily diet—is a surefire losing strategy. Forget it. As the Buddhists say, there is only now. The longer you wait to face your stress, the longer you hope and pray that it might miraculously go away, the tougher it gets to regain control over your life. Take action! How? I have two simple yet profound formulas that will teach you the techniques you need to conquer stress.

This is your wake-up call.

The First Formula: Conquering Stress

Formula #1 lays out the big picture. It encourages taking the high road in terms of caring for your health. It focuses on one of the fundamental, point-blank principles of previous chapters:

Nutrition makes you feel good; stress makes you feel bad.

Concentrate on this breakthrough concept: To create a mind-set that overcomes stress, make the Wellness Process a top priority. Wellness, with a capital W, stands for happiness, fulfillment, and vibrant health. The path, the process, to Wellness gives you the strength to get the better of oxidative stress—one road leads to the other.

Wellness comes from integrating mind, body, heart, and soul. It means you are fully alive, operating at peak capacity. The pure glory of being impassions you. Take a look at this true-to-life equation:

$$\textbf{Wellness} = \frac{\textbf{Nutrition}}{\textbf{Stression}}$$

Nutrition is the ongoing act of self-enrichment. Its opposite, stression, is the ongoing act of self-depletion. Once you understand and accept this simple formula, the key to overcoming stress will be revealed.

I call this equation the Wellness Index: It can be used to measure your level of Wellness—meaning your level of nutrition in relation to your level of stress. Take these three high-stress scenarios as examples:

- High-performance nutrition keeps your Wellness level competitive and buffers high stress.
- Average nutrition makes it difficult to sustain Wellness. Stress will have the upper hand.
- Poor nutrition debilitates your Wellness level. In the battle for control of your body, stress is winning. You are losing.

In other words, when confronted with high stress levels, **the only way to achieve Wellness is through high-performance nutrition.** High-performance nutrition puts oxidative stress in its place.

If we study this simple formula more closely, we can draw some interesting conclusions about the relationship between oxidative stress and high-performance nutrition:

- The greater your level of physical fitness and nutrition, the greater your Wellness Index, regardless of your level of stress.
- The better, and longer, you nurture yourself, the lesser the impact of stress and the more it takes to throw you out of balance.
- The higher your nutrition levels, the better prepared you are to handle sudden, unforeseen, stressful events.
- The more oxidative stress you suffer from, the more vulnerable you are to the effects of poor nutrition, and the greater your need for high-performance nutrition.

High-performance nutrition empowers you. It is the antidote for oxidative stress. It gives your body the tools to squarely face stress, instead of relying on anything else—junk food, liquor, workaholism, recreational drugs, sex— as an emotional crutch.

HIGH-PERFORMANCE NUTRITION MATTERS

High-performance nutrition isn't just about diet. It's about healing your whole self. Anything you do to enhance your well-being is nutritious: Important components include, for example, good friends, good humor and good sex in addition to good food. Self-respect is very nutritious. Engaging in your own personal relationship with divinity as you perceive it is spiritually nourishing. The point being, high-performance nutrition encompasses emotional, mental, and spiritual, as well as physical, health.

High-performance nutrition makes life work right. Family, home, and career all function harmoniously. Each day holds purpose and promise. Be it through professional accomplishments or personal relationships, you are making a difference in other people's lives. Your spiritual and secular selves are in balance, and your positive mental attitude empowers every aspect of your existence.

Stressition, on the other hand, sabotages. Instead of thriving, you're barely surviving under the weight of all that oxidation. A self-abusive, undisciplined lifestyle gradually takes it toll, resulting in disruptive personal relationships and counterproductive behavior on the job. That's apparent on the outside. On the inside, target organs start to fail. Your energy level drops, and eventually illness sets in.

Three out of every four Americans—a shocking 75 percent—are afflicted with either cancer or heart disease in their lifetime. That statistic alone should be compelling enough to get us to pay attention to high-performance nutrition.

Conclusion: Overcome stress with high-performance nutrition.

The Second Formula: How to Achieve High-Performance Nutrition

From this point forward, for the purposes of *Food Swings*, when I refer to high-performance nutrition, I will be speaking specifically about diet. Formula #2 details how to achieve it.

High-performance nutrition is about knowing what to eat, and then making sure you eat it. The combinations vary per individual, but all high-performance foods are **fresh**, **pure**, and **whole**. **High in fiber**, **low in fat**, and **chemical-free**. To receive the full benefits of high-performance eating, you need to know *how* to eat *what* is best for *you*. You must honestly account for your food choices and eating habits. To achieve high-performance nutrition, swear by these three action steps:

- **Step 1**   **Change your attitude: select for smartness rather than taste**
- **Step 2**   **Acquire nutritional know-how: learn what to eat**
- **Step 3**   **Take consistent positive action**

Remember the three steps through their key words:

Attitude, Know-How, Action=Transformation

STEP 1: Change Your Attitude: Select for Smartness Rather Than Taste

It's time to take a new look at your relationship to food. We've been raised in a culture that values instant gratification over long-term benefits. When we eat, we think only of the immediate, sensual appeal of food, and not of the negative effects it may ultimately have on our health. Formula #2 demands that we re-prioritize our food choices, so that we select items based on their nutritional value, rather than their initial taste or their emotional, mommy-daddy appeal. This is smart and savvy eating.

It's also, at least at first, a challenge.

The good news is, smart eating can still be satisfying. It doesn't turn food into a grim obligation. A smart diet includes tasteful food that is clever enough to also be healthy. In fact, there is even such a thing as *gourmet* smart food.

Smart food heals and energizes. It has a positive impact on mind and body in both the sensory short term and the physiological long term. Put more simply, it's good now and later!

All Formula #2's first step requires is a slight shift in outlook: Eat to live, don't live to eat.

Mommy-daddy diets aside, we all have the need to be emotionally nurtured by our food. Looking forward to mealtime is a natural instinct, and dining together is an important part of social communication, be it between friends, a couple, or a family. But, just as in any other relationship, there's a difference between equality and dependency. Smart food ultimately empowers you, giving you the **energy advantage** on life's many playing fields—on the job, in love, at home. It builds your brainpower, enabling you to achieve more professionally. It boosts your self-confidence, because it makes you feel so darn good.

FREE YOUR MIND

You, and only you, own your attitude. You have the ability to change your eating habits. The "glass is half empty/glass is half full" philosophy can be applied to any area of thinking, including your outlook on food.

Doctors of preventive medicine learn that attitude is the deciding factor in a patient's behavior, and many experts believe that **habits are active states of attitude**—ingrained ways of being created by repetition. In other words, your attitude about eating and your actual eating habits are inextricably interwoven. Thought leads to action. The same thoughts about food, repeated regularly over the course of many years, eventually become automatic, almost unconscious, responses. The same stimuli arouse your impulse to eat, and you feel powerless to resist.

Exercise buddies Jean and Karen have different eating habits. After their morning jog, they pass by a pastry shop. Jean can't wait to reward herself with a treat. Within seconds, she succumbs to the bakery's sweet aromas and buys the brightest goodies on display. Karen sees and smells the exact same items, but she is not lured by the fragrance of fresh brewed coffee and sugary donuts. She's anticipating the fruit salad and bowl of muesli and soy milk that await her at home.

Karen, of course, has the smart food attitude. She won't sabotage her daily jog for an eclair. She respects her body and wants to look and feel her best. It took her a little time: Like most of us, she was raised on the SAD—**S**tandard **A**merican **D**iet. But in her mid-twenties she decided that fitness and health came first, and devoted some attention to nutrition and the healing arts. At this point, she is not even attracted to food that is not good for her. She knows that sugary desserts and caffeinated coffee drain her energy, and she finds fruit salad more appealing, even on a visual level. Jean, on the other hand, feels she is at the mercy of croissants and cappuccino.

The difference between the two women is attitude. Karen's attitude is positively disciplined, and as a result her eating habits are healthy. Over time, she has established a routine that is in her own best interest. She is in control.

Jean, however, has been doing the donut-and-coffee routine for fifteen years now. She considers her morning ritual a reward, and she looks forward to it. The sugar and caffeine serve as a pick-me-up for the busy day ahead. Although she has a good attitude toward her job and her daughter, she doesn't think as highly of herself or, by extension, her diet. She lacks discipline, and indulges her impulses. She wants her diet to be exciting, and believes she is entitled to unlimited pleasures from her most preferred foods.

There's a conspiracy at work in the food industry. Truly. No, it's not as if the captains of leading companies hold secret meetings in smoke-filled backrooms, but the food industry capitalizes on the average American's stress level and his or her need to use food for recreation. We've all been programmed to eat what is popular, and the most popular items are those that are most heavily advertised and most readily available. Choosing natural plant foods over their commercialized competitors is a challenge. Defying the majority and breaking free from family habits can be stressful and confusing. Some people may see your positive choice as a criticism of their own diet, and ostracize you for changing. It requires character and courage.

Jean is confused. She probably doesn't realize she's in the danger zone, on a collision course with burnout. She looks at food as a crutch to get her through a tough day, while Karen thinks the day itself is its own reward. She wants to maximize her relationship with each day through high-performance nutrition.

LYIN', CHEATIN', LOWDOWN, DIRTY, GOOD-FOR-NUTHIN'. . .

Let's say you're single, and you meet someone you find physically attractive, so you embark upon a relationship. But let's also say that this certain someone doesn't tell the truth and cannot be trusted. He or she takes more than he or she gives, and steals your valuables behind your back. How long would you stay in that relationship? What is the benefit of continuing it?

The same holds true for food selections. Anti-nutrients may have some superficial sizzle, but they're bad for you. They're all flash, no substance, and they often stress you out.

We humans are blessed with free will. We can change our attitudes about the emotional and entertainment value we attach to food. It is within our power to select wholesome nutrition that is still enjoyable. Ask yourself, what's holding you back?

You may disagree with my nutritional posture. You may protest that filet mignon, chicken enchiladas, and chocolate chip ice cream make you feel so good, you couldn't stand to live without them. I have heard many a patient rationalize, "I eat okay. Take away my favorite foods, and what else is there to live for?" And I know that these favorites sensually stimulate and emotionally appeal to your appetite. But there's a price to pay when you invest in a losing strategy.

Just like any other bad relationship, eating for pleasure rather than wellness will ultimately let you down. The best foods, like the best friends, are in it for the long haul.

In twenty-five years of practice, the most common justification I hear from my patients for persisting in their poor diet habits is this: Eating better is *boring*. But that's The Conspiracy at work! It has brainwashed the American populace so that they can't recognize the flavor of smart food. High-performance nutrition is colorful and fragrant. Fruits, vegetables, grains, and beans can be aesthetically appealing. And by using a variety of herbs and seasonings, you can prepare smart food to fit your tastes. To tempt your palate, think of: tomato-basil-mushroom pasta; rich minestrone soup; thick guacamole, chunky salsa, and creamy hummus dips; nutty soy spreads; veggie pizzas; plus an assortment of Indian and Chinese dishes.

Here's what I tell my patients: As long as your senses are intact, you can have an exciting, uplifting, emotional relationship with smart food. Deprivation is a relative concept. If you were blind, and could not see food, you would be visually deprived. If you were afflicted with a cancer of the throat or tongue, and had undergone surgery that eliminated your ability to taste or swallow, you would be sensorially deprived. But as long as you can smell, see, touch, taste, chew, and swallow, then you are equipped with the necessary tools to build an appetizing yet healthy connection to whole food.

One final point about attitude: When you change the way you think about eating, you don't just change your appetite for *food*. There's a ripple effect that impacts your appetite for *life*. Great health transforms everything, from your performance in sports, to your stamina when the flu fells everyone else at the office, to your energy level at the end of the day when your kids need help with their homework. By feeding your body, you're also feeding your soul.

As you develop a taste for smart foods, I guarantee that you'll also become emotionally attached to them. In fact, you'll *take pride* in them. After all, they're the real thing—wholesome, fresh, colorful, tactile. They have not been pressed, bleached, or chemically altered.

Another positive side-effect of high-performance nutrition is the way, over time, it reprograms your body's chemistry. After eating natural, wholesome foods for a few years, you'll find that, health concerns aside, the traditional SAD diet actually *tastes* terrible—to you, the person who once swore undying devotion to Philly cheese steaks! I've had patients who've slipped, and they often complain of feeling nauseated and dizzy after indulging in what used to be their favorite junk foods. Similarly, when you first begin to introduce smart food into your diet, a glass of fresh squeezed carrot juice may upset your digestive system, since your body has become so accustomed to soda. Taste buds are creatures of habit, adjusting to what is most familiar.

Apply the benefit-to-risk ratio when making your smart food selections. Choose produce with the most benefits and least risks. For example, The Conspiracy would like you to believe that eggs are the perfect protein. But eggs are sky-high in cholesterol and extremely mucus-forming. They put the consumer at risk for everything from the common cold to respiratory problems to clogged arteries. In other words, the risks of egg consumption far outweigh the benefits, especially when you can substitute scrambled tofu, sautéed lightly in olive oil with onions and mushrooms, and gain the equivalent protein value without the fat, cholesterol, or phlegm.

Select for effect—that's another skill of the nutritionally inclined. With a little practice, you'll be able to gauge the way certain foods make you feel. Pay attention to your body's reaction: Do certain items have a soporific effect? Give you a headache? Disrupt your sleep? Whenever food has negative repercussions, your choice is sense-oriented instead of smart-oriented.

Chronic dieters joke "a minute on the lips, an eternity on the hips" when trying to dissuade themselves from some fatty temptation. But the damage caused by anti-nutrients is much more than cosmetic. Is it really worth ruining your health just to satisfy your ingrained, gluttonous lust?

STEP 2: Acquire Nutritional Know-How: Learn What to Eat

A clear-cut nutritional philosophy enables you to choose smart foods. If knowledge is power, then an understanding of high-performance nutrition leads to the stockpiling of anti-aging antioxidants. There is a direct connection between smart food consumption and antioxidant accumulation.

Later in this chapter, I'll present specific high-performance food choices, but first, let's quickly recap the relationship between antioxidants and free radicals.

Oxidative stress refers to the damage caused by free radicals. Free radical damage can occur in the body's tissues at the cellular level, and can ultimately lead to target organ failure. The cumulative effect of oxidative stress is aging and illness. The degree to which the body is damaged by free radicals is determined by the amount of antioxidants on hand to fight back. Antioxidants defend your body against damage from free radicals.

ANTIOXIDANTS: THE ULTIMATE WEAPON

Antioxidants inactivate free radicals, thereby protecting the body from the adverse effects of alcohol, caffeine, sugar, and other negative food choices. The body produces its own antioxidants, but high-performance nutrition increases the supply. It also strengthens the immune system.

Conversely, poor nutrition releases free radicals into the body. High-fat, artificially flavored foods introduce chemical toxins into the system. Because they increase oxidative stress, free radicals are also known as pro-oxidants. Instead of protecting, they attack nerves, arteries, joints, and organs. Compare:

FREE RADICALS	ANTIOXIDANTS
promote oxidation	prevent oxidation
found in anti-nutrients	found in the body's immune system and in whole food nutrients
accelerate damage	detoxify, rejuvenate, and regenerate

Consider the example of atherosclerosis: When you overeat saturated fats and other oxidative-stress-causing anti-nutrients, they release chemical toxins that line the arterial walls. The toxins eventually accumulate into a plaque that obstructs the flow of blood to vital organs. Hardened arteries decrease circulation to the heart, brain, and kidneys, and can result in such fatal illnesses as cardiac arrest and stroke.

The more antioxidants and fewer free radicals in your diet, the better your health.

PREMIUM GASOLINE

The best foods for your body are high-fiber, low-fat and chemical-free. They contain the highest concentration of nutrients and, by extension, antioxidants. The list below differentiates between some common smart and poor food choices—you'll recognize many of the latter from the previous chapter.

HIGH-QUALITY FUEL	LOW-QUALITY FUEL
(high in antioxidants)	**(high in free radicals)**
fresh fruit	butters, ice cream, and dairy
fresh vegetables	heavily salted foods, saturated fats
whole grains	commercial breakfast cereals
legumes and beans	beef and pork protein
freshly squeezed juices	coffee and soda
sprouts	refined white sugar
nuts and seeds	refined white carbohydrates

Before you can begin experiencing the benefits of high-performance nutrition, you have to know what to eat. Let's start with the rules:

THE SEVEN RULES OF HIGHLY EFFECTIVE EATERS

1. TAKE FULL RESPONSIBILITY FOR EVERYTHING YOU EAT.
2. SELECT FOOD ON THE BASIS OF QUALITY.
3. SELECT ALKALINE FOOD OVER ACID-FORMING FOOD.
4. SELECT HIGH-FIBER OVER LOW-FIBER FOODS.
5. BALANCE YOUR DIET WITH PROPER PROPORTIONS FROM THE FOUR ALTERNATIVE FOOD GROUPS.
6. SIMPLIFY.
7. SELECT COMPLETE PROTEINS.

Rule 1: Take full responsibility for everything you eat

When it comes to your health, you are in the driver's seat, and you select your body's fuel. Top-grade fuel helps an engine to run efficiently; low-grade results in deficiencies; too much floods the system.

Face it. Food is everywhere—at wedding receptions, corporate functions, Little League games. It's inescapable. So don't let situations get the best of you. And don't use them as an excuse. Just because, for example, you go to the movies, it doesn't mean you have to eat a tub of popcorn. At the point of purchase, you are in charge.

Eating is a daily, multidimensional experience, incorporating everything from your family background to your financial status to your emotional fragility. Acknowledge its complexity, end the blame game, and stop pointing fingers at your mate, friends, and family whenever you indulge. Educate yourself, respect yourself, and learn to trust in yourself. The only person who can make certain you eat well is you.

Once you feel comfortably in control of your ability to resist the top ten stress food categories, take yourself to the next level of nutritional empowerment and proactively choose high-performance items that promote antioxidation.

Rule 2: Select food on the basis of quality

High-performance nutrition is a powerful form of preventive medicine. Whole foods provide the body with an abundance of healing nutrients, and experts agree that a natural, pure, balanced diet is essential for sustaining health. But the majority of Americans select food not on the basis of quality, but on the basis of convenience and emotional comfort. In 1995, a large supermarket chain in San Diego released the results of a survey it had conducted: The store had asked 1,000 shoppers what criteria they applied when loading up their shopping carts. Not surprisingly, most people considered their best food buys the ones that were the least expensive, the easiest to prepare, and the most emotionally appealing. This, of course, is why advertisers emphasize the sensual aspect of food: steaks are *juicy*, chicken breasts *tender*, sour cream *zesty*, and so on.

Although food is often at the center of social activities, you can exercise good nutritional judgment without inconveniencing or insulting others who might not share your high-performance preferences. The same foods hold different meaning to different people, so it's important to respect their right to their own nutritional choices, even if you think they are abusive. Be tolerant, take it easy, and teach by example. When you are looking and feeling great, friends will eventually want to know why.

But while being humble about your nutritional know-how, stand up for your beliefs. Your friends and family should be equally respectful of your own food choices, and shouldn't bully you for breaking free from the herd. The purpose of a communal meal is the interaction. Whether or not everyone eats the same thing should be a secondary consideration. So don't buckle under social pressures and compromise to appease anyone else.

Follow these four principles to guarantee that you select foods on the basis of quality:

- ■ **Principle 1** Select fresh food over devitalized items
- ■ **Principle 2** Select whole, unprocessed food over fragmented, processed products
- ■ **Principle 3** Select pure food over chemical toxins
- ■ **Principle 4** Select natural over synthetic foods

Or, further abbreviated, remember the four positive principles through their key words:

Fresh, Whole, Pure, Natural

Principle 1: Select fresh food over devitalized items

At least half of your diet should be comprised of fresh, raw, living food. As I'll explain in subsequent chapters, fresh foods abound with antioxidizing enzymes and phytonutrients. Fresh fruits and vegetables have the power to heal, restore, and sustain your energy level. They promote a highly efficient metabolism, nurture the liver, stimulate the glands, and regulate hormonal balance so that you can burn fat fast. They accelerate the conversion of other foods into energy. Devitalized, dead items, such as slaughtered meats and canned goods, are much more difficult to metabolize.

Principle 2: Select whole, unprocessed foods over fragmented processed products

Processing, refining, and storage techniques depreciate the nutritive value of food (think about how long that can of green beans may have been sitting at the back of the pantry shelf, and the varying temperatures it must have withstood). Refined sugars and carbohydrates offer only empty calories. For example, in the refining process of a whole grain such as wheat, both the bran of the outer coat and the germ at its center are removed. This depletes the wheat of more than 20 vital nutrients, including vitamins B and E and calcium. When four of the 20 nutrients are returned to the denatured carbohydrate, packagers label it "enriched." Why mess with Mother Nature's brilliant handiwork to begin with? Select whole, unprocessed foods, and avoid refined, processed substitutes.

Principle 3: Select pure foods over chemical toxins

The SAD diet is plagued with toxic chemicals that send oxidative stress levels skyrocketing. Canned fruits and vegetables, prepackaged microwave meals, TV dinners, delicatessen meats, frozen foods, and instant breakfast cereals all commonly contain an assortment of chemical fertilizers, artificial flavorings, insecticides, chlorinated pesticides, additives, sodium nitrates and nitrites, monosodium glutamate (MSG), and colored gums and dyes. Poisonous preservatives, chemical sprays, and injected hormones invite allergies and decay. Polluted, drugged, contaminated foods weaken the immune system and increase the risk of cancer. Not exactly an appetizing thought, is it?

Principle 4: Select natural over synthetic foods

The more natural the food, the higher its nutritional value; select organically grown items whenever possible. Today, most soil is chemically treated to the point that such healing minerals as selenium and vanadium are eliminated, but organic foods are raised in soil that's rich with natural fertilizers. This enables them to retain the highest content of trace minerals, vitamins, and enzymes. If organic food is not yet readily available where you live, don't worry too much about it. You can still achieve nutritional excellence with fresh, whole, and pure foods.

Rule 3: Select Alkaline Food over Acid-Forming Food

The issue of alkaline versus acidic foods will come up often when you're deciding which proteins work best in your high-performance diet. The Conspiracy wants you to associate meat, fish, fowl, eggs, cheese, milk, and dairy with protein, but these animal products actually introduce acidic toxins into your system. The resulting acid overload increases the rate of oxidation, including that of cholesterol into artery-blocking plaque build-up. A vegetarian diet, however, promotes an alkaline biochemistry that the body much prefers. Blood, serum, and other vital fluids are all optimally alkaline, operating at a pH level of 7.4. (A pH of 7 is neutral; above is alkaline, below acidic.) The kidneys, in their ongoing attempt to flush out toxins, strive to maintain a dominantly alkaline balance.

Second to food allergies, over-acidification is the most undiagnosed condition I want to challenge. Excess acidity increases the risk of atherosclerosis, multiple sclerosis, cancer, and Parkinson's disease. It is the root cause of liver and kidney disease. It upsets the digestive system, aggravating the esophagus, stomach, and pancreas. By imbalancing spinal and joint fluids, it precipitates the onset of arthritis, rheumatism, fibromyalgia, and osteoporosis. It even triggers common skin problems such as eczema and fungal infections.

Take note of some of the most common alkaline and acidic foods:

HIGHLY ALKALINE FOODS	HIGHLY ACIDIC FOODS
Almonds	Beef protein
Broccoli	Chicken protein
Carrots	Eggs
Green, leafy vegetables	Fatty Fish (e.g., sardines)
Papaya	Organ Meats
Potatoes	Pork Protein
Soybeans (e.g., tofu)	Shellfish (e.g., crab)
Sunflower Greens	Smoked Fish (e.g., herring)
Watermelon	
Wheat grass	

Rule 4: Select high-fiber over low-fiber foods

This one is a no-brainer. In the medical community, it's undisputed that a high-fiber diet is far superior to a low-fiber one. Fiber does more than regulate your intestinal tract and increase the efficiency of your digestive and waste disposal systems. It also lowers cholesterol, improves the absorption rate of vital nutrients, and helps prevent breast, colon, and rectum cancers. Fiber deficiency, on the other hand, invites diverticulitis, spastic colon, and irritable bowel syndrome.

Check out the fiber content of these common foods:

FOOD	SERVING SIZE	GRAMS OF FIBER
Meat and Dairy		
Chicken	any amount	0
Dairy	any amount	0

FOOD	SERVING SIZE	GRAMS OF FIBER
Eggs	any amount	0
Fish	any amount	0
Red Meat	any amount	0

Grains, Pastas, Tofu and Tempeh

Brown Rice	½ cup	2.4
White Rice	½ cup	0.8
Couscous	½ cup	0.5
Millet	½ cup	3.5
Polenta	½ cup	2.0
Quinoa	½ cup	5.0
Spaghetti	½ cup	2.0
Tabbouleh	⅔ cup	1.0
Tempeh	⅓ block	8.0
Tofu	⅕ block	1.0

Cold and Hot Cereals

Corn Flakes	¾ cup	2.7
Grape Nuts™	1 oz	1.8
Millet Rice	¾ cup	3.0
Multigrain	⅔ cup	4.0
Oatmeal	½ cup	7.7
Puffed Rice	1 cup	1.0
Wheaties™	1 cup	2.6

Breads

Bagel	1	0.6
Bran Muffin	1	2.5
Focaccia	1 slice	1.0
Multigrain	1 slice	2.0
Rye Bread	1 slice	0.9
Spelt	1 slice	0.9
Wheat Bread	1 slice	1.4
Wheat Tortilla	1 tortilla	2.0
White Tortilla	1 tortilla	0.5

FOOD	SERVING SIZE	GRAMS OF FIBER
Beans, Peas, Legumes		
Chickpeas	½ cup	6.0
Green Beans	½ cup	2.1
Kidney Beans	½ cup	5.8
Lentils	½ cup	3.7
Lima Beans	½ cup	4.4
Pinto Beans	½ cup	2.5
Split Peas	½ cup	2.5
Vegetables		
Artichoke	1 large	4.5
Asparagus	½ cup	1.0
Avocado	½ cup	2.8
Beets	½ cup	2.5
Broccoli	½ cup	2.2
Carrots	1 med.	1.5
Cauliflower	½ cup	1.0
Corn on the Cob	1 med.	5.0
Cucumber	½ cup	0.4
Mushrooms	½ cup	1.5
Potato (w/skin)	1 med.	2.5
Romaine Lettuce	1 cup	2.0
Salsa	2 tbsp	1.0
Sea Nori	1 sheet	1.0
Spinach	½ cup	7.0
Steamed Veggies	1 large plate	6.5
Tomato	1 med.	1.5
Tomato Sauce	½ cup	2.0
Zucchini	½ cup	1.8
Fruits		
Apple (w/skin)	1 med.	3.5
Cantaloupe	¼ melon	1.0
Figs	1 med.	2.0
Grapefruit	½	0.8
Orange	1 med.	2.6

FOOD	SERVING SIZE	GRAMS OF FIBER
Prunes	3	3.0
Raspberries	½ cup	4.5
Watermelon	1 slice	2.8
Nuts and Seeds		
Almonds	10 nuts	1.1
Peanut butter	2 tbsp	2.0
Sesame butter	2 tbsp	2.0
Sunflower seeds	1 cup	2.0
Snack Foods		
Corn tortilla chips	1 oz.	2.0
Popcorn	1 cup	1.0
Potato Chip	1 oz	1.0
Garden burger	1 patty	5.0
Multigrain waffle	1	2.0
Wheat crackers	4	1.0

Rule 5: Balance your diet with proper proportions from the four alternative food groups

Contrary to popular opinion, the four food groups are NOT meat, dairy, white bread, and dessert. For optimum nutrition, adhere to these four alternative food groups:

I.	Natural, Simple Carbohydrates (e.g., fresh fruits and vegetables, and their natural juices)	50%
II.	Whole, Complex Carbohydrates (e.g., whole grain breads, pastas, and cereals; brown rice; potatoes)	20–25%
III.	Non-Animal Proteins (e.g., beans, legumes, tofu, tempeh, and veggie burgers)	15–20%
IV.	Natural Fats (e.g., monounsaturated and unsaturated oils; avocado; unsalted seeds, nuts, and nut butters)	10–15%

A peak-performance diet combines a high percentage of simple and complex carbohydrates with a moderate amount of non-animal proteins and a small quantity of natural fats.

Rule 6: Simplify

You would expect it to be simple to simplify your diet. And you're right. It is. As you become better educated about nutrition, determine which foods are in and which are out. Then stick to it. Simple, yes? Although it may sound deceptively straightforward, setting boundaries for yourself makes a big difference. Eliminating anti-nutrients simplifies your diet. Committing 100 percent to your nutritional plan simplifies the decision-making process every time you go out to a restaurant. Of course, as you discover new, alternative, whole food options you'll want to incorporate them *into* your plan. But decide now what gets *ousted*.

Rule 7: Select Complete Proteins

By combining fresh, raw foods with complete, non-animal proteins, you can consistently create high-performance meals. To get you in the habit of the maximum protein-fresh food mix-and-match, I've outlined some sample meals:

BREAKFAST

A fresh fruit salad (1–1½ cups) with any one of the following will turn breakfast into a complete protein meal:

1. 1 oz unsalted almonds with 2 oz low-fat granola
2. 1–2 tbsp nut butter (unsalted almond butter is preferred) with 2 oz granola
3. 1–2 slices sprouted seven-grain bread with 1–2 tbsp nut butter
4. 1 oz almonds with a ½ to 1 cup serving of seven-grain cereal: oatmeal, millet, bran, cream-of-rye, or cream-of-wheat
5. 1–3 oz mixed nuts

LUNCH

Depending on your level of activity, lunch can be light, moderate, or more substantial:

Lightweight Lunch

Option 1

A fresh fruit salad (1–1½ cups) with any one of the following will make lunch a complete protein meal:

1. ½ cup low-fat soy cottage cheese
2. ½ cup non-fat soy yogurt
3. 1–3 oz nuts and seeds

Option 2

Adding any one of the following combinations to a leafy green chlorophyll salad (1–2 cups) will make lunch a complete protein meal:

1. raw carrots, peas, mushrooms, and 2 tsp sunflower seeds
2. ½ cup steamed carrots, ½ cup steamed peas, 8 medium mushrooms, and 2 tsp sunflower seeds
3. 1 cup steamed green vegetables in season with 2 tsp sunflower seeds
4. or, on the side of the salad, avocado inside a heated corn tortilla for a guacamole taco

Dr. Meltzer's Lightweight Fruit Smoothie:

For a third lunch option, toss a seasonal fruit salad (1 cup) into the blender with: 1–2 tbsp Re-Vita*; 1 tbsp brewer's yeast; 1 tbsp bee pollen; 1 banana; 1–2 cups of fresh-squeezed fruit juice; 1 tbsp of almond butter or 10 unsalted, roasted almonds; and ice.

*See Resource

Welterweight Lunch

A leafy green chlorophyll salad plus any one of the following will make lunch a complete protein meal.

Mixed into the salad:

1. ½ cup of tabbouleh with 2 tsp sunflower seeds
2. ½ cup of tofu with celery, onions, and tomato
3. ½ cup of eggless potato salad with 2 tsp sunflower seeds

Two teaspoons sunflower or sesame seeds in the salad, with an 8–10 oz serving of any one of the following soups on the side:

4. lima bean
5. bean-vegetable
6. split pea
7. mushroom
8. carrot-onion
9. lentil
10. potato-leek, with ½ cup of soy cottage salad or ½ cup eggless tofu salad

On the side of the salad:

11. guacamole (made from half an avocado) on carrot or celery sticks
12. vegetarian taco: fresh, raw or steamed vegetables inside a warm corn tortilla; avocado optional
13. avocado sandwich: half an avocado spread on 2 slices of sprouted seven-grain bread
14. Mideastern garbanzo spread (hummus—2–3 tbsp) with whole-wheat pita pocket bread

Heavyweight Lunch

A leafy green chlorophyll salad plus any one of the following will make lunch a complete protein meal:

1. half an avocado on sprouted seven-grain bread; mixed vegetable soup (8 oz) on the side
2. whole wheat pita stuffed with avocado, tomato, sprouts, and onions; mixed vegetable soup on the side
3. lentil soup with 1–2 slices sprouted seven-grain bread
4. guacamole with vegetable bean soup
5. corn tortilla or whole wheat chapati stuffed with guacamole (no cheese); mixed vegetable soup on the side
6. quesadilla: corn tortilla with rennetless or soy-based cheese; mixed vegetable soup on the side
7. falafel: whole wheat pita stuffed with garbanzo-bean patty
8. veggie burger: mushroom, soy, lentil, garbanzo, or tofu burger on whole wheat bun; or without bread, but with vegetable soup on the side
9. split pea soup with 1–2 slices sprouted seven-grain or whole wheat pita bread
10. bean vegetable soup with 1–2 slices sprouted seven-grain or whole wheat pita bread

DINNER

For complete protein dinners, combine a leafy green chlorophyll salad with one option from any of the following six categories (recipes can be found in the back of the book):

Complete Soybean Combinations

1. scrambled tofu with vegetables
2. scrambled tofu with ½ cup brown or wild rice
3. tofu chop suey with vegetarian egg rolls
4. tofu lasagna (use your favorite lasagna recipe, but substitute soy cheese for cheese and scrambled tofu instead of meat)
5. vegetable casserole (soybeans and vegetables on brown rice)
6. soy burger on whole grain bun
7. tempeh burger on whole grain bun
8. soy cheeseburger on whole grain bun

9. soy grits with ½ cup of cooked brown rice and ½ cup of soy milk
10. whole grain pasta with tofu and fresh tomato sauce

Complete Bean Combinations

1. organic tostada: corn tortilla, ½ cup cooked beans (kidney and pinto), sprouts, tomato
2. falafel: ¼ cup garbanzo beans made into a patty combined with mushrooms, onions, green bell pepper, and sesame seeds, with or without pita bread
3. hummus Lebanese dip: ½ cup cooked garbanzo bean spread, ½ slices whole wheat pita
4. beans and rice: mung beans, adzuki, lima, kidney, and pinto beans with brown or wild rice, ½ cup each
5. vegetarian enchiladas, burritos, or tamales

Complete Soup and Grain Combinations

1. lima bean vegetable soup with 1–2 slices whole grain bread
2. lima bean vegetable soup with brown rice
3. split pea soup with ½ cup brown or wild rice
4. split pea soup with 1–2 slices whole grain or whole wheat pita bread
5. minestrone bean vegetable soup with ½ cup brown rice
6. minestrone bean vegetable soup with 1–2 slices whole grain bread
7. mushroom soup with whole grain pasta noodles and fresh tomato sauce
8. vegetable soup with whole grain pasta noodles and fresh tomato sauce, mixed with scrambled tofu

Complete Lentil Combinations

1. lentil mixed vegetable soup with raw or sautéed mushrooms
2. lentil-mushroom-vegetable casserole; 2 tsp sesame or sunflower seeds in the salad
3. lentil-sesame-nut roast
4. lentil soup with 1–2 slices whole grain or whole wheat pita bread

5. lentil soup with ½ cup brown rice or millet
6. lentil burger on whole wheat bun

Complete Pea Combinations

1. steamed peas, steamed carrots, 1 baked potato; 2 tsp sesame or sunflower seeds in the salad
2. vegetable casserole; 2 tsp sesame or sunflower seeds in the salad

Complete Dairy Combinations

Use soy or rennetless cheese:

1. vegetarian lasagna
2. vegetarian pizza
3. vegetarian enchilada
4. eggplant parmesan
5. zucchini-rice casserole (with or without cheese)

GENERAL GUIDELINES

In general, keep the following guidelines in mind when combining foods

Maintain an alkaline-to-acid ratio of 3:2; preferably 2:1

Maintain a raw-to-cooked ratio of 1:1, and up to 2:1

Eat at least 25–30 grams of fiber daily

Balance colors: Prepare visually appealing high-performance meals

Flavor: Use herbs to make food taste great

Step 3: Take Consistent Positive Action

In our super-commercialized society, we are constantly bombarded with misleading information from the profit-focused food industry. The majority of advertised food products are inferior at best, and institutionalized nutrition—school lunch programs, hospital food, and the like—fail the American public. Save yourself with high performance nutrition. Consistent proper, positive food selections start the journey to self-health.

Depending on your individual schedule, some days you will have to plan out or prepare your meals in advance. Anticipate your needs and take appropriate action. Again, consistency is crucial. Make smart eating a habit, like putting on your seat belt each time you get in your car. High-performance foods can't help you unless you eat them!

Systematically undereating smart foods at regular intervals in a relaxed manner will change every aspect of your life. In the next chapter, I'll set forth a series of rules that will help you stick to a high-performance nutrition plan. They'll teach you how to put your education into action, by choosing smart foods that produce beneficial food swings.

CHAPTER 6
THE GOLDEN RULES FOR SMART EATING.

Positive thought leads to positive action. Retrain the brain to relish whole foods, and the body will soon follow suit. Think about the energy advantage high-performance nutrition will afford you. Think about the increased life span. Think about the smaller dress and pants size. Then put those thoughts to work! Follow my Golden Rules for smart eating and you'll soon be nutritionally empowered. Sure, it requires some discipline, but if you deliberately repeat the same positive actions, eventually they'll become dominant lifestyle habits—the norm, not the exception, and as natural to you as breathing. **Taking control of your thoughts and food-moods leads to nutritional consistency.**

The Golden Rules give you the guidelines necessary to consistently eat smart. They're positive thoughts put down on paper. Memorize them. Copy them yourself, then carry around the page in your wallet, tape it to the kitchen refrigerator, post it on your computer at work. The only way to achieve high-performance nutrition is through consistent life-affirming dietary decisions.

Several characteristics define our eating habits:

- *what* you eat
- *when* you eat
- *how much* you eat
- *how fast* you eat
- *your attitude* before and while you eat
- *your posture* when you eat
- *your level of relaxation* when you eat

Identifying these characteristics—running down that checklist—every time you eat will teach you to distinguish healthy habits from unhealthy ones. As you become more aware of your negative behaviors, it will become more difficult for you to allow yourself to continue them. My Golden Rules will clear up any confusion about what constitutes a positive food choice.

EMOTIONAL HUNGER

The true purpose of eating is simple: We need vital nutrients to fuel our biological systems. That's it. But over time, food has taken on all sorts of secondary objectives. We eat certain foods based on our ethnic heritage, or to mark a specific situation. For example, as children, we begin to associate cake with birthdays from the very first time we go to a party. By far the most destructive, self-defeating reason we eat is to fill an emotional void. **We use food to lift our mood.**

Emotional hunger is possibly the biggest obstacle on the road to high-performance nutrition. Most of us know smart food is better for our bodies than fast food, so why do we still succumb to the lure of steak, cake, and take-out? The answer has to do with the emotional distractions that accompany stress. When we're anxious, depressed, or under pressure, our level of contentment is threatened. Instead of facing the situation, we often feel an overpowering urge for the quick fix mommy-daddy foods can be counted on to provide. We know in our heads that this kind of false comfort has negative consequences, but our emotional needs overrule logic.

When Doug is feeling frustrated at the end of the day, he believes he deserves a few quesadillas before bed. As far as he's concerned, the amount of food he's already consumed for dinner is irrelevant, because he's focused on consoling, rewarding, and entertaining himself. Nourishment does not factor into the equation. Nor does his obesity: At six feet and 312 pounds, he's at least a hundred pounds overweight. Doug is a coronary waiting to happen, but the food fix comes first. Because his EKG is normal, his physicians do not feel compelled to prescribe a healthier diet.

Marcy also indulges at night. Her drug of choice is ice cream. She desperately wants to lose weight but, like Scarlet O'Hara, she always vows to think about it "tomorrow." Today, she's under too much stress at work. Deep down, Marcy knows that her stress feeds her negative food swings, which in turn feed her stress, but she can't muster up the self-control needed to stop the vicious cycle.

Emotionally comforting foods like quesadillas and ice cream exploit the hand-to-mouth reflex. They trigger a primitive reaction, a basic instinct, one that precedes our socialization with fork and knife. To resist, it's vitally important to adopt a system, one that can adapt to the adversity of everyday life and fortify you when you're most vulnerable—whether at a restaurant or party, away on business or vacation, or, most important, when you're tired and blue. Put your faith in my foolproof system and learn to master your binges, cravings, and out-of-control emotional hunger. Eating strictly for emotional pleasure is a losing strategy. With a positive attitude, the proper foods, and the Golden Rules at your disposable, you can win.

The Golden Rules are geared toward achieving high-performance nutrition, of course, but they come with an added bonus: They'll teach you to resolve emotional distractions and dilemmas, instead of pacifying them with junk food.

THE STREATEGY

When first addressing the Golden Rules, keep an open mind and a light heart. If you think of your mommy-daddy diet as the enemy, naturally, the enemy is not going to be pleased to encounter a worthy opponent. Stress, cravings, and compulsive habits will have to come face-to-face with the Golden Rules. The more ingrained your negative food habits, the harder it will be, at first, to adopt the rules. Recognize the challenge, and don't get discouraged early in the game!

Dr. Meltzer's Golden Rules

THE PRE-MEAL StrEATegy

1. EARN YOUR MEALS.
2. RELAX FOR AT LEAST FIFTEEN MINUTES BEFORE EACH MEAL—MEDITATE OR PRAY.
3. DRINK FRESHLY SQUEEZED FRUIT JUICE FIFTEEN MINUTES BEFORE BREAKFAST.
4. DRINK FRESHLY SQUEEZED CARROT OR OTHER VEGETABLE JUICE FIFTEEN MINUTES BEFORE DINNER.
5. CREATE A SPIRITUAL, HEALING AMBIENCE AT MEALTIME.
6. COMMIT YOURSELF TO HIGH-PERFORMANCE NUTRITION.

THE MEALTIME StrEATegy

1. RELAX WHILE YOU'RE EATING: FIND YOUR RHYTHM.
2. ALLOW YOURSELF AT LEAST A HALF HOUR TO SIT DOWN AND GET COMPLETELY INVOLVED WITH YOUR MEAL.
3. SCHEDULE YOUR MEALS AT REGULAR TIMES THROUGHOUT THE DAY.
4. EAT WHEN YOU ARE HUNGRY, DON'T WHEN YOU'RE NOT, AND UNDEREAT IN THE SPIRIT OF MODERATION.
5. SUBSTITUTE INTIMATE CONVERSATION AND GOOD COMPANY FOR OVER-INDULGENCE.
6. DON'T EAT WHEN YOU'RE NERVOUS.
7. CHEW SLOWLY, ONE BITE AT A TIME.
8. APPRECIATE AND ENJOY YOUR FOOD: KEEP A POSITIVE MENTAL ATTITUDE.
9. POSTURE COUNTS: SIT UP STRAIGHT.
10. BE SOULFUL WHILE EATING.

THE POST-MEAL StrEATegy

1. KEEP MENTALLY AND PHYSICALLY ACTIVE.

The Pre-Meal Streategy

1. Earn Your Meals

Earning your meals is about deserving your meals. The body is designed to work hard and stay in shape. In fact, neglecting your body could be considered a form of disrespect, even self-abuse. Earning meals teaches us to value our body and understand its relationship to food. It teaches us not to take meals for granted.

To earn your meals, exercise before most, if not all, of them. It's essential to get your day off to the right start by working out before breakfast. Optimally, exercise precedes dinner, too. In the morning, get the blood pumping with at least twenty minutes of cardio or aerobic exercise. In the evening, condition muscles and joints through at least twenty minutes of yoga, gym work, Tai Chi, or a brisk walk. There are four distinct benefits to working your body before eating. Exercise:

- regulates your metabolism
- regulates your appetite
- tunes up your digestive system
- maximizes your assimilation of nutrients

Earning your meals regulates your metabolism. Exercise before meals prepares your body to efficiently convert nutrients into fuel. It charges up your digestive batteries. Your activity level is directly linked to your metabolism, or body chemistry, and, by extension, the rate at which you burn fat. Regular exercise gives your body a foundation, a base, for effective fat-burning. After you have expended a significant amount of energy, your body will want to replenish it with nutrients. Consistent daily exercise, preferably before meals, is the most direct way to make your metabolism calorie-efficient. It trains the body to extract just enough fuel from the minimal amount of smart foods.

Earning your meals regulates your appetite. Exercise is a key to permanent weight loss. When you refresh your mind and body before eating, you work up a natural appetite, and can avoid nervous overeating. Many experts believe that a regular fitness routine releases endorphins—feel-good natural neuropeptides—into the bloodstream, and that their presence contributes significantly to a prolonged positive mental outlook. Exercise is a mood elevator that's always going up. It's a natural antidepressant. And when you feel content, calm, and centered, it's easier to eat well.

Earning your meals tunes up your digestive system. Exercise is also a predigestive aid. Working out coordinates your circulatory, respiratory, and digestive processes. It activates the digestive enzymes and prepares the liver to perform at its peak potential.

Earning your meals maximizes your assimilation of nutrients. Again, by shifting all the metabolic machinery into high gear, exercise increases the amount of and rate at which the body absorbs and utilizes nutrients.

2. Relax for at Least Fifteen Minutes Before Each Meal—Meditate or Pray

Relaxation is like the flip side of exercise: It's just as important to condition your mind as your body before a meal. To downshift from the exercise-induced endorphin high, take fifteen minutes to meditate or pray. You need more than just a moment to really unwind. America was founded on the Puritan work ethic; to this day most of us are afflicted with relaxation-deficit disorder and choose to ignore it. But, like exercise, relaxation before eating increases the assimilation of nutrients and aids the digestive system. Also like exercise, relaxation keeps you calm enough to control your appetite.

If mind and body are in a state of balance, digestive enzymes, nerves, and hormones can cofunction efficiently. When nervous, many people speak of "butterflies in the stomach" or complain of a tummy ache. When relaxed, the opposite is true. Meditation or prayer promotes liver, pancreatic, and intestinal wellness.

I also prescribe active relaxation as a way to reduce anxiety. ("Active relaxation" is not an oxymoron: There's a big difference between collecting your thoughts in fifteen minutes of silent meditation and slouching on the couch watching television for four hours.) Stress impairs the body's ability to digest food, which can lead to fermentation and the accumulation of toxic residue. Not good. Setting aside some quiet time before each meal helps to reduce your level of stress and thereby increase your digestive capacity.

Ideally, I recommend that patients go for the full mind-body combo before both breakfast and dinner, although I realize it isn't always a practical option. I call the morning routine of aerobic exercise and meditation, in fifteen-to-twenty-minute segments each, the **Sunrise Cleanse**. The Sunrise Cleanse refreshes the mind, strengthens the body, opens the heart, and stokes the soul—all within the first hour of the day. The **Sunset Recharge** does all of the same things, before dinner.

Think of how powerful these first two rules are. For example, how often would you eat if you only ate when you were relaxed and had worked out first? On the other hand, eating when you are both physically and mentally uptight can compromise your digestive efficiency and invite dysfunctional food swings. Physical and psychological stress weaken your resolve. Nervous energy turns to negative food choices as an outlet for emotional tension.

Danger: KNOW WHEN NOT TO EAT: Do Not Eat When Nervous

The nervous system strongly influences appetite. It's easier to face down emotional hunger and make smart choices when you're calm. Subsequently, wholesome choices prove their worth by prolonging your sense of well-being. Suddenly, you start to hear your body telling you what it needs. Eventually, overindulging just doesn't feel right anymore, not even in those once-beloved gluttonous moments.

3. Drink Freshly Squeezed Fruit Juice Fifteen Minutes Before Breakfast

Start the day right by drinking freshly squeezed fruit juice after exercising and before you meditate during your Sunrise Cleanse. I recommend juices from fruits that are in season: Watermelon in summer, apple juice in fall, and orange or grapefruit juice from winter into spring. You don't have to strain half a watermelon every June morning, but do make sure the juice you buy is labeled "fresh-squeezed," not from concentrate. Drinking juice fifteen minutes before breakfast gives your digestive enzymes a gentle wake-up call while you're meditating. By the time you eat, your digestive juices will be at the ready for fruits and nuts.

4. Drink Freshly Squeezed Carrot Juice Fifteen Minutes Before Dinner

The same principle holds true for the Sunset Recharge. Just as you'll precede your fruit meals with fruit juice, you'll precede your vegetable-based meals with fresh vegetable juice. Carrot juice is especially effective, but carrot-celery or carrot-celery-beet juice also work well. As with fruit juice in the morning, vegetable juice in the evening—after you exercise and before you meditate or pray—arouses your digestive enzymes. The alkaline in carrot juice helps to balance the chemicals at work in the stomach and liver, thereby improving digestion, assimilation, and waste disposal.

5. Create a Spiritual, Healing Ambience at Mealtime

Although our stressful culture doesn't usually value them as such, meals ought to be one of our most respectful daily rituals. They are an opportunity to self-nourish, self-nurture, and self-express. Eat your meals in the most serene, aesthetically soothing setting you can create at the moment. Ideally, have flowers or plants nearby. In the morning, if possible, sit in a sunlit room—or, if weather permits, eat outside, on the porch or in the yard. Fresh air and a scenic view have a calming effect on mind and body. At night, lower the lights and spark a few candles for a warm ambience. Avoid eating in the car, in front of the television, or when you're talking on the phone. Think of your dining area as a sanctuary, a place where you can seek refuge from all the chaos of the outside world. Don't bring that chaos into the sanctuary by, for example, listening to the radio or reading the newspaper while you eat.

6. Commit Yourself to High-Performance Nutrition

It might sound obvious, but regularly reaffirming your commitment to high-performance nutrition helps to strengthen your resolve. In this regard, the pre-meal streategies of meditation, a healing ambience, and reaffirmation go hand in hand: They're all ways of clearing the mind and keeping you centered. Your eating habits can only be as good as your nutritional philosophy. So repeat after me:

High-performance nutrition provides life-promoting nutrients.

Remind yourself that smart foods feature essential antioxidants and enzymes. Conversely, the chemically processed foods that characterize the SAD diet are devitalized—the life has literally been taken out of them.

Regularly recommitting yourself to high-performance foods helps you to resist the temptation to cheat on your diet—and, by doing so, to cheat your body out of necessary nutrients. By affirming your vow to eat well, feel good, and look great, you encourage your habits to follow your intentions.

You make the effort to get to work on time each day, or pay your bills when they're due, or mail holiday cards each year. These are things you do for your own, but also for others', sake. I'm asking you to be selfish. To do something just for you. Not for your boss, or the telephone company, or your Great-Aunt Hilda. Make the commitment to yourself, and yourself alone, to positive eating habits. Commitment leads to consistency, consistency leads to success, and frankly, you're worth it.

The Mealtime StrEATegy

1. Relax While You're Eating: Find Your Rhythm
AND

2. Allow Yourself a Half Hour to Sit Down and Get Completely Involved with Your Meal

Relaxation is a prerequisite to high-performance nutrition. When nerves, stomach, intestines, and liver are in synch, the body is best prepared to digest. The Sunrise Cleanse and Sunset Recharge are focused on relaxing you before eating. It's equally important to maintain that calm composure throughout the meal itself. Without a full relaxation response at mealtimes, you can fall prey to certain digestive dysfunctions.

Slow Down with Slow Food

Slowing down enables you to get the most out of your meals. Slow foods are those that take a little time to prepare, a little time to consume, and, once swallowed, are fully digested for all their nutritional potential. They're the opposite of fast food. Brown rice with tofu and green vegetables is an example of a slow meal. Chicken in a bucket with a side of fries is not.

In addition to being good for you, slow food can also be quite romantic. Allow yourself to enjoy the ritual of preparing slow meals by turning off the ringer on the phone, turning on some soothing music, or listening to the sounds of silence. Relax.

Thirty minutes is the minimum amount of time it takes to effectively stimulate the pancreatic enzymes responsible for digesting most nutrients. Designating at least thirty minutes to meals gives your body a solid opportunity to assimilate nutrients. It also gives your mind and soul a chance to unwind. At first, you may protest that you can't afford the time. The key is to make your meals a priority, as important to you as, for example, your favorite television programs.

3. Schedule Your Meals at Regular Times Throughout the Day

Timing your meals is one of the secrets of clinical nutrition. Done properly, it can greatly improve the effectiveness of your diet. How do you get your timing right for breakfast, lunch, and dinner?

Breakfast: When it comes to breakfast, the earlier the better—after the Sunrise Cleanse. Plan to eat breakfast by 8:30 A.M. in the warmer months and by 7:30 during the shorter days of winter.

Lunch: Eat lunch between noon and 1:30. Later lunches, or skipping lunch, can throw off your timing for the rest of the day.

Dinner: Dinner is best metabolized right after sunset (and the Sunset Recharge!), before it gets dark, so keep an eye on the light. Eating too late in the evening can disrupt your sleep by overtaxing your digestive organs, and drain you of valuable energy the next day. Keep your evenings event-filled and socially rewarding, so that you feel less of a need to depend on dinner for emotional fulfillment.

For a three-meal day, work within this time frame:

- Breakfast: 6:30—8:30 A.M.
- Lunch: 12:00—1:30 P.M.
- Dinner: 5:30—7:30 P.M.

The importance of biorhythms is often overlooked, but your digestive organs function best as creatures of good habits. Eating at set intervals establishes order and continuity in the liver, biliary, stomach, and intestines. It also regulates waste elimination. Spacing meals about six hours apart allows your body to engage in the entire cycle of nutrient absorption and waste elimination, then recover in time for the next feeding. Consider the opposite, but more common, scenario: Many of us eat breakfast late, and lunch too soon afterward, so that the body's processing of the first meal is interrupted by the arrival of the second. By the afternoon, we're stuffed and sluggish, and postpone dinner until late in the evening. And that's not even considering what it is we're actually eating.

A regular meal schedule also helps you to stay in control of your lifestyle. Knowing when you plan to eat each day helps you to avoid many pitfalls, such as resorting to candy for an energy rush in the late afternoon because you've somehow neglected to have lunch, or loading up on carbohydrates too close to bedtime.

When you find yourself out of sync and off schedule—particularly when you've eaten a late breakfast—skip the next meal to get back in rhythm.

4. UNDEREAT IN THE SPIRIT OF MODERATION: Eat When You're Hungry, Don't When You're Not.

Often, we eat whatever is in front of us without thinking much about it.

It never even occurs to us that we don't *have* to finish the pizza, or get to the bottom of the bag of chips. Instead of stuffing your system with the mommy-daddy foods you think it wants, listen to your body, fuel it with what it needs, and stop eating once you've had enough.

Undereating defines the line between a balanced diet and indulgence. It allows your body to get the most out of the food you eat, because by under-feeding it, you're giving the digestive system a few key fossil-fuel ingredients to focus on—not a quagmire of anti-nutritional gunk to slog through. If you're assigned a project at work, you do a better, more thorough job when you can really focus your attention on it. But if you're overwhelmed with a million other responsibilities, it's likely that the best you'll do with the new assignment is just manage. The body is no different.

Undereating emphasizes putting down the fork and getting up from the table before you feel completely full, when you still have an appetite and could probably still eat some more. Because nearly everybody overeats, prac-ticing undereating will help you to eventually find a middle ground, one where you're eating just the right amount. If you think you might be overeat-ing, you probably are. Stop right that second! Don't take another bite.

The body is equipped with an internal alarm that goes off when the brain realizes you've had too much to eat or drink. The problem is, many of us have learned to tune out this alarm. In order to tune back in, it's important to relax and listen. Many of us are actually frightened by the prospect of hearing what our body has to say—we stuff ourselves to silence it, afraid to face the truth-telling. But even if we've been abusing it, our body is always on our side! It's our greatest ally. Just as in any other healthy relationship, we have to be able to communicate with it.

Think of moderating what you eat as the microcosmic equivalent of bal-ancing what you do. Just as balance is essential to personal and profession-al success, so, too, is moderation essential to dietary success. Mind and body prosper when fueled by the proper proportions of smart, slow food. And it's an incredibly liberating feeling when you can comfortably, confidently say no to that extra serving.

Sally on the Graveyard Shift

Sally, a nurse, had been working the graveyard shift at her hospital for the past seven years. She'd punch in at 11:00 P.M., punch out at 7:00 A.M., five days a week. Sadly, she'd become so obese that she actually preferred to work these desolate hours. She reasoned that as long as she worked while the rest of the world was sleeping, fewer people could see just how heavy she'd gotten.

Sally had the proverbial "pretty face," but, at 5'8" and 205 pounds, she was about 40 pounds overweight. She'd become so isolated and self-loathing that it took the constant prompting of her best girlfriend to get her to my clinic. With a blank look on her face, the first thing Sally said when she met me was, "I have no willpower, Doctor Meltzer. I enjoy eating all the time, under any circumstance."

"When do you eat?" I inquired.

"Oh, maybe two to three times . . ."

I was about to ask her just what she ate those two to three times a day when she continued, ". . . two to three times in the morning, two to three times each afternoon, and two to three times at night."

"So you'd estimate you eat up to nine times a day?" I asked, trying to downplay my distress.

"Actually, I'm so stressed out that I eat whenever I get the opportunity."

In Sally's world, "opportunity" equaled any time food was in sight. On her way to work each night, she'd stop by one of the many fast-food chains. At the hospital, she made frequent visits to the cafeteria and hit the vending machines in between. On her way home in the morning, she looked forward to pancakes and eggs at one of the local diners before she went to bed. Eating was the most important, most interesting, thing in her life.

I took a thorough medical history. In the process of describing her health, Sally revealed how lonely and socially frustrated she was at the age of 41. Although I sympathized, I also gently explained to her that her emotional attachment to food was not only hurting her health but also compounding her personal problems. I outlined a specific diet, and told her about the benefits of undereating in the spirit of moderation. Sally protested that she was too overweight to be able to accurately assess when she'd had enough. But I assuaged her fears.

"It's simple," I told her. "When you're uncertain if you're eating too much, ask yourself, 'Am I eating too much?' Then listen to your body for the answer."

Although the prospect of "talking" with her body terrified her, Sally took my program to heart. She soon found herself satisfied by a salad and a cup of soup, when previously she'd gone through three to five plates per meal. Sally learned to say no.

Do Not Eat When You Are Not Hungry

It's okay to skip a meal once in a while. If you are diabetic or suffer from a metabolic condition such as hypoglycemia or hyperthyroidism, then it's best that you not miss any meals. But the rest of us should not force ourselves if we are not hungry. Sometimes, at our regularly scheduled breakfast hour, for example, we might feel like reading, writing, doing some yoga, talking with a loved one, whatever. The emotional balance that these sorts of activities bring is in keeping with smart eating, so trust what your body tells you. Ask yourself if you want to eat. The answer may legitimately be no. In fact, it can be good training to condition yourself to only eat when you are genuinely hungry—it prepares you for times when you may actually have to skip a meal because smart foods are not available. Have a salad, a smoothie, a fruit cup, or some herbal tea. Then, even if your natural appetite returns between regularly scheduled meals, hold off until the next designated eating time. This way, you'll stick to your daily agenda.

5. Substitute Intimate Conversation and Good Company for Over-Indulgence

They say laughter is the best medicine. Companionship at mealtime is good for the soul, and it actually curbs your appetite by shifting the focus from eating to socializing. There are times when it is quite healing to enjoy breakfast or lunch alone, in a relaxed natural environment. But at dinner, permit yourself some esprit de corps by spending time with loved ones, friends, and family. Eating together with intimates promotes emotional balance which, in turn, keeps emotional hunger at bay. The celebration of people takes precedence over the celebration of the palate.

6. KNOW WHEN NOT TO EAT: Don't Eat When You're Nervous

Avoid eating when you're upset, anxious, or stressed. The Sunrise Cleanse and Sunset Recharge will go a long way toward calming your nerves and keeping you in a balanced yet vital state. But if the pre-meal workout and meditation doesn't adequately alleviate your agitation, avoid eating until you can determine how to resolve the emotional conflict. Eating when upset invariably sets a dysfunctional food swing in motion. Knowing what *not* to eat and when *not* to eat it is just as important as the more positive counterparts. In the next chapter, I'll go into more detail about how to prevent dysfunctional food swings.

7. Chew Slowly, One Bite at a Time

Extend the relaxation principle by maintaining a slow, steady pace when you eat. Remember that meals are opportunities to put your busy schedule on pause. They may be your only chance during an otherwise hectic day to take a break from responsibilities and chores. Pace yourself for a thirty-minute meal the same way you'd pace yourself for a three-mile run. Start slowly, one bite at a time. Don't inhale (or, as we say in California, "hoover") your food. Fully taste each forkful you put in your mouth. Relish it. If it helps, eat one food at a time: For example, don't mix carrots and broccoli in the same bite.

Start with crispy, raw salads. Chew thoroughly, so that you grind out the water in the leafy greens. Crunch seeds and nuts. Masticate. The activity of the jaw reveals a lot about a person. Some people chomp nonstop, jowls jiggling, from the beginning to the end of a meal. Hurried, high-speed jawing raises the issues of hidden stress, sexual frustrations, or other emotional inhibitions.

Dave's Ultimatum

Dave was plagued by so much gas that his odor-assaulted wife gave him two alternatives: See a nutritionist or sign a divorce agreement. (Luckily for him, he was living in a no-fault state.) In our consultation, I explained to Dave that there were many different causes of *flatus*—the clinical term for wind. Potential culprits included: food allergies; explosive food combos; intestinal fermentation of undigested protein or starch; nervous eating habits; dysbiosis (a bacterial deficiency); excess protein; excess bread; insufficient pancreatic enzymes; colon dysfunction; emotional stress; and poor assimilation of foods. I took on the role of detective, determined to get to the root of the problem.

A preliminary nutritional survey came up blank. In fact, I was impressed with Dave's educated food choices. I realized I'd have to investigate further.

That evening, my family wanted to eat at a favorite Italian restaurant, so at about 7:00, we sat down to dinner. Call it coincidence, luck, or fate, but

Dave and his disgruntled wife were sitting just a few tables away. I couldn't help but observe my patient in action. In the amount of time I'd ordinarily allot to a dinner salad, Dave had downed his entire meal. Mouth, teeth, and jaws were in high gear. He gulped forkful after forkful.

It was clear to me then that Dave had acquired a common eating habit. He would work hard all day, and when it came time for dinner, all he wanted was to be left alone to wolf down his food. It was his way of recovering. At first, he was surprised by my prescription: eat slowly, after having exercised and meditated before meals. But within a few short weeks, he had bid good riddance to his chronic gas—and his marriage was back on track.

8. Appreciate and Enjoy Your Food: Keep a Positive Mental Attitude

Ours is such a prosperous society that we often take food for granted. We no longer value it for its vital properties. We think of it instead as a form of entertainment. "Starvation in the midst of plenty" describes the dilemma of having many food choices yet still suffering from a lack of true nutrition. "Overconsumption malnutrition," a qualitative deficiency state in which the "victim" suffers not from poverty or famine but from overeating empty calories, characterizes the SAD diet. It's a shame.

Try to recognize the real, earthy magnificence of whole food, and the important role it plays in your life. Treat it with respect. Instead of pausing to appreciate nature's great gifts, most of us rush through our meals. Saying grace aloud, or silently affirming, or simply holding hands, are all ways of expressing gratitude for the aesthetic, emotional, and nutritive value of food. You can also show your consideration for food by selecting organically grown produce and preparing wholesome dishes.

During our first consultation, many of my patients state, with embarrassment and resignation, "I love to eat." Of course you love to eat! Everyone does. Eating is one of the great joys in life. We should not deny ourselves this pleasure, or be ashamed of it. We just need to shift the balance back to where it belongs, so that food fulfills its maximum potential to nourish, without being an emotional crutch. To start, ask yourself what foods you find exciting. If the answers fall into any of the junk categories outlined in Chapter 4, then there's a glitch in the system. Don't despair. Recognizing the problem is always the first step toward fixing it. Once you've identified your food traps, you know to expect them, and can learn how to dismantle them. Over the course of your life, many negative influences have conspired to get you addicted to your poor diet. Your parents may not have consciously intended for you to use food as a substitute for love, but they did encourage it every time they rewarded or placated you with sweets. On the other hand, The Conspiracy, as I refer to it (only half-jokingly!), most certainly did want to hook you, and it spends millions of dollars in advertising each year to keep you on the junk. You've been brainwashed. Now it's time to take control of your own deprogramming.

From a physiological standpoint, enjoying what you eat leads to a more complete release of digestive enzymes and, consequently, a more complete assimilation of nutrients. When you are in an anxious mood, your digestive efficiency is decreased, because your body is diverting its attention elsewhere. It can't focus, for example, on the regular removal of waste because it's too busy working to combat the agitation of the nervous system. Without getting into too much medical detail, all sorts of digestive ailments—from stomach ulcers to spastic colons—are caused at least in part by imbalanced emotional states. Dave's flatulence demonstrates this.

Attitude affects appetite, so turn on your food. You know that food turns you on, but what do you think your energy does to it? Remember that when you subscribe to high-performance nutrition, both you *and* your food are alive. A positive mental attitude brings out the positive principles in food. A healthy emotional connection to your diet expedites your ability to convert dietary nutrients.

9. Posture Counts: Sit Up Straight

Your posture makes a difference at mealtimes. Circulation to the digestive glands improves when you are seated because, due to gravity, blood pools in the digestive system. In fact, I encourage fledgling yogis to sit cross-legged, lotus or semi-lotus style, at a low table. The position is optimal for digestion, because it allows blood to wash over the digestive organs and liver. But, except when eating at exotic eastern restaurants, this position is often socially impractical, so the next best option is to sit in a chair that offers firm back support. Avoid hunching your spine. And one exception: Sitting in your car—even if you're sitting up straight!—and stuffing down take-out while driving does not count as a smart food move. (Not to mention that it may be hazardous to your fellow motorists!)

Standing up while eating is a bad habit of our hectic age, and does not work to our benefit. When we stand, blood drains from the stomach and pools instead in the veins of the legs, where it doesn't do us any digestive good. Furthermore, standing while eating encourages myriad negative food swings. Prime example? Raiding the refrigerator. How many times have you opened the refrigerator door *not* to take out whole food items needed to prepare a planned meal, but just to check out your snacking options? You don't really know what you're looking for when you open the door, you're just hoping to find something to munch.

If it's not a designated mealtime, get out of the kitchen.

10. Be Soulful While Eating

Acknowledge the divine in yourself and your diet. In a manner that corresponds to your own personal belief system, bless your kitchen and dining room, and recognize them as healing centers. Most of us think of soul food as a Southern variety, deep-fried and smothered with gravy, but when you stop to consider it, high-performance, alkaline, antioxidant whole food is the real soul food, because it promotes life.

Acknowledge the privilege of being alive. Converting living food into fuel for work and play is no less than a divine process. Many religions use food as a metaphor for life, and it is central to sacred rituals. Our body *is* a temple, our own personal cathedral, and we have the honor of maintaining it. Every day offers us a chance to come fully to life through our choice of food. Stress and negative food swings prevent us from prospering in our own private Eden.

The Post-Meal Streategy

The point of the post-meal streategy is simple: Move on. Do not make a career out of your meals. After you eat, especially in the evening, take a brisk, fifteen-minute walk. Otherwise, it's very easy to get drowsy after dinner. This also holds true for late afternoons at the office. If you eat at your desk and then go right back to business, without ever having gotten up, changed locations, or moved about, I guarantee your head will begin to droop. Those whose jobs keep them on their feet during the day, whether it's because they're store clerks or schoolteachers or hospital doctors, often succumb to the post-supper couch-potato syndrome. I understand the exhaustion, but sinking into the sofa after dinner stalls the metabolism. After you've enjoyed a smart meal, move on to a physically and mentally stimulating activity.

PART 2

PREVENT DYSFUNCTIONAL FOOD SWINGS AND TAKE CONTROL OF YOUR DIET

BY NOW, you should have a better understanding of the different memories and emotions you attach to specific foods. That's your individual relationship. But the country as a whole is suffering from a dietary epidemic: I call it *appetitis*—an inflammation of the appetite.

To cure appetitis, it's important, first and foremost, to be able to tell the difference between hunger and appetite. Next, pinpoint your particular variation of the disease: I describe eight of the most common manifestations, including bingeing and "food-on-the-brain" syndrome. The R.R.I.E.A. technique, which I outline in Chapter 8, explains how to counter the onset of appetitis, and Top Ten lists of the most energizing, sexiest, most tiring, and best anti-depressing foods provide you with a kitchen arsenal of nutritional aids.

CHAPTER 7

HOW TO PREVENT
DYSFUNCTIONAL FOOD SWINGS

On an intellectual level, you've come to understand the power that stress has over your eating habits. You've itemized your mommy-daddy diet, recognized Emotional Tension, and memorized my Golden Rules. Now it's time to put your new nutritional philosophy to the test. Understanding the nature of your negative food swings will help you to disarm them forever.

In our self-aware society, we've all become familiar with the term "dysfunctional." It's the psychologist's way of saying that something "sort of works"—but in an adverse, damaging manner. A dysfunctional family, for example, is still a family. But its problems prevent it from being a healthy, happy, communicative unit. Dysfunctional behavior is often so deeply ingrained that it's difficult to see the destructive patterns; the hurtful cycles are enacted again and again. Dysfunctional food swings wreak havoc on not only your emotional well-being, but also your physical health.

Dysfunctional food swings are not good for you. They disrupt your lifestyle, and they create and keep re-creating emotional instability. In fact, dysfunctional food swings can cause you bodily harm. Dysfunctional food swings feed themselves into a viscious cycle of self-abuse: Bad Moods → Bad Eating Habits → Stress, Fatigue → Bad Eating Habits → Bad Moods.

What I call *oxidative food swings* characterize our high-stress culture. In the standard American diet, overeating anti-nutrients at irregular intervals is so commonplace that, as with any other dysfunctional pattern, we hardly even recognize what we're doing is dangerous. Dysfunctional food swings deceive. We think they make us feel good, and initially, from a purely sensual standpoint, they do. In the meantime, their long-term impact on our body is 100 percent bad. And the general sluggishness and malaise they create weakens willpower. The next time we're under stress, we turn right back to the bacon double cheeseburger.

Dysfunctional food swings feed off stress, and stress feeds off dysfunctional food swings.

It's a murderous merry-go-round.

WEEDS IN THE GARDEN

Out-of-control overeating, compulsive bingeing, mindless snacking, or late-night indulging promote rotten general health, the three degrees of burnout, accelerated aging, serious illness, and, eventually, death. Like weeds, these dysfunctional food swings spread stealthily, choking off the roots of healthy plants and ultimately consuming an entire garden. Disruptive food swings feed on this stress, and stress feeds on moodiness and abusive eating habits. In turn, dysfunctional mood swings are known to trigger more stress. Take a look at how oxidative stress turns into a repetitive cycle of destructive eating habits and destructive food swings.

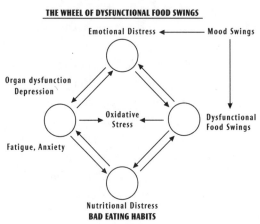

THE WHEEL OF DYSFUNCTIONAL FOOD SWINGS

For the vast majority of Americans, dysfunctional—or oxidative—food swings seem almost unavoidable. In the morning, you're late for work and have no time to make breakfast, so you stop at a local deli to get a bagel with cream cheese and a coffee, light, two sugars, to go. At lunch, you're too busy to leave the office, so you order in a pizza, buy a soda at the vending machine, and down them at your desk while returning phone calls and e-mails. By night-time, you're too exhausted to cook anything that requires more effort than pushing the buttons on the microwave. The next day, you get up and do it all over again.

What can be done to stop the cycle of abuse?

Like any other medical condition, dysfunctional food swings can be approached in two ways. We can prevent them or we can treat them. Prevention is always preferable. Given the choice, why develop bad habits to begin with? Often, bad habits become so ingrained on so many levels—physical, mental, emotional—they're almost impossible to break. Smoking is the most obvious example of this syndrome. Physically, a smoker becomes addicted to nicotine. Mentally, a smoker may associate the habit with certain characteristics s/he admires, such as sophistication. Emotionally, smoking, like junk food, exploits the hand-to-mouth reflex. When a smoker attempts to quit, s/he finds himself fighting the habit on many different fronts. It's an uphill battle.

In upcoming chapters, I'll address how to treat specific dysfunctional food swings. For the moment, however, let's talk about prevention.

AN OUNCE OF PREVENTION . . .

. . . is worth a pound of cure. There's a lot of wisdom in that homespun adage. The active, intentional prevention of illness keeps disease from occurring. **You get it before it gets you.** Compared to the effects of even the most advanced medical techniques, staying healthy far outweighs any benefits of being treated. Curing illness involves restoring health to diseased tissues. It's much better never to damage the tissue at all.

By the same token, it is better never to permit dysfunctional food swings. They serve little purpose. At best, they help you to recognize the components of your particular mommy-daddy diet, and once you've experienced the negative results one too many times—you're tired of being tired, for example, or frustrated by your expanding waistline—then dysfunctional food swings can serve as a call to action.

I branched out into preventive medicine because I'd become intrigued with the idea of maintaining mind and body in a proactive state that would fight off illness. After four years of medical school and three as a surgical resident, I was aggravated, even bored, by all the different, newly developed, incredibly costly methods of bailing out an abused body. Late one night in the operating room, I experienced an epiphany. I was working as a surgical resident with a team of University of California surgeons pioneering innovations in liver transplants. The patient, a 55-year-old male, had terminal, end-stage cirrhosis caused by excessive alcohol consumption. We'd spent fourteen hours in the operating room, and had to return to the OR at midnight because complications—internal bleeding—had appeared. As a group of physicians, nurses, and in-house staff worked feverishly to save the man's life, I found myself wondering why my work was always concentrated on crisis resolution. Over the course of the operation, one thought recurred to me. It circled my mind like a mantra: "There's got to be a better way." And then it came to me. It was as if another voice had heard me thinking, and replied: "There is. Prevent it."

I can still remember that stormy February night when the seeds of my career in preventive medicine were planted. Since then, I have learned some simple yet profound lessons:

What is the best way to prevent disease?

The best way to prevent disease is to be well. It's basic logic: If you have wellness, there's no room for illness. The two can't coexist simultaneously in the same body.

What is the best way to prevent dysfunctional food swings?

The best way to prevent dysfunctional foods swings is to follow *healthy* food swings. That's right. The best way to prevent negative food swings is to experience the benefits of *positive* food swings. The right habits prevent the wrong habits. Relaxed, nutritious eating habits prevent stress-related eating habits.

Furthermore, the prevention of stress-related dysfunctional food swings is an essential part of any preventive medicine plan.

It all fits together quite naturally.

PRIMARY FOOD SWINGS BUILD THE FOUNDATION

Food swings describe the impact different foods have on the mind and body. **Smart, high-performance foods "swing," or shift, your metabolism in an affirmative direction.** The regular selection of superior foods, combined with sensible eating habits, leads to the establishment of a foundation—a foundation of nutrition that will support the body as it faces new challenges each day. Just as disease is often degenerative, declining by degrees of illness, so, too, is wellness progressive. Healthy habits have a cumulative effect. Put simply, if you follow healthy habits for one day, your body benefits for that day alone. But if you follow healthy habits for a year, and then are faced with, for example, a flu virus, your body can call to the front an entire twelve months worth of wellness to combat the intruder. Make sense?

Primary nutritional food swings, then, are those first positive food swings needed to build the foundation for the long term while keeping you energized in the present moment. By providing your metabolism with the right nutrients, they begin the process of revitalizing it.

Food swings expose the personality of your eating habits. Because whatever you eat has to be metabolized, whatever you eat causes a reaction, or swing, in your body chemistry. Actions—eating—demand reactions—digestion, absorption, expulsion, etc. Depending on what you imbibe or ingest, the body reacts differently. It calibrates its response based on when you eat, what you eat, how much you eat, and your mood while eating. It's fine-tuned, so that each food choice and eating habit directly relates to the resulting emotional state and energy level. Just as you'd expect from a brilliant, self-sustaining machine.

PRIMARY FOOD SWINGS AT THE PUMP

Primary food swings have an immediate positive impact. They lift and stabilize moods, increase energy, and calm nerves. Put more eloquently, they are curative, restorative, and resurgent. They relieve stress—and prevent dysfunctional food swings.

Pretend you just purchased a brand new SUV for your family. And let's make the dreamworld more interesting by stipulating that you only get one car per lifetime, but it has the potential to last as long as you do. To power your new vehicle, you have three choices of fuel at the gas station:

- The gas at Pump #1 will protect the engine and keep the car running well for its life expectancy.
- The gas at Pump #2 will keep the car running, but you can expect mechanical malfunctions about twenty-five years down the road. The lower quality of fuel will gradually corrode and oxidize the engine.
- The gas at Pump #3 mixes the high-quality and low-quality fuels offered at the previous two pumps.

Which fuel would you choose?

The lower quality of fuel from the second and third pumps will result in premature degeneration of your vehicle. You may have plenty of good years to start, but sooner or later your prized automobile will turn into a jalopy and you'll wish you'd only ever used the gas in the first pump.

After all, you only get one car for your whole life.

As a doctor, I often wonder why anyone would choose the dietary equivalents of pumps #2 or #3, when we have pump #1 at our disposable. I understand that food frequently fills many other, non-nutritional needs, and that it's human nature to crave immediate gratification. But don't we all want to live life to the fullest (especially considering the alternative—loss of resilience and death without dignity)? The SAD diet may momentarily placate the terrors of our daily chaos, but cancer, stroke, heart disease, arthritis, diabetes, and multiple sclerosis are a hundred times more stressful than a bad-hair day. Smart food has the now-and-later benefit of helping us deal with our present-day stress while preparing our bodies to fight off future illnesses. Dumb food does exactly the opposite. It adds to our daily stress, and makes us all the more susceptible to disease.

By the way, in addition to adding weight to your own body, you also make the commercial food industry fat and happy when you eat junk food.

PRIMARY FOOD SWINGS PREVENT DISEASE

Undereating antioxidant nutrition in a relaxed manner at regular intervals establishes primary food swings and reinforces your self-control. Consistent primary food swings are the best type of preventive medicine. They're habit-forming, but in a positive way. Master your eating habits, and you master your food swings.

Primary nutritional food swings turn on the self-regulatory switches that keep the body in balance. They rejuvenate and protect. They are anti-oxidant, and therefore anti-aging. Dysfunctional, oxidative food swings, by contrast, accelerate the aging process.

Primary food swings involve eating foods rich in true nutrients and antioxidants.

Oxidative food swings involve eating foods high in anti-nutrients and pro-oxidants.

When primary food swings dominate oxidative food swings, you reinforce the preventive foundation. Primary food swings are forward-moving. Their process includes experiencing, enjoying, understanding, and sustaining smart food selections. In previous chapters, we've discussed foods to avoid, foods to choose, and the Golden Rules of Smart Eating. The next step is to apply this knowledge. Direct your attention to creating and maintaining a balanced, mutually supportive relationship between your body and your diet. Make it a priority. Practice.

THE TWO DEGREES OF PREVENTION

Primary nutritional food swings directly relate to primary preventive care. Primary prevention addresses a patient's habits, evaluates his or her risks for disease, then initiates a plan to reduce and/or eliminate these factors. In other words, primary prevention calls for active participation in a self-directed wellness program.

Secondary prevention focuses on detecting disease in its early stages. Mammograms, Pap smears, and X rays are all examples of secondary preventive action. As the involvement of doctors, nurses, and technicians might indicate, secondary prevention is more passive than primary prevention. At the secondary level, things are done *to* you by medical professionals. At the primary level, you have a hand in your own health.

THE SEVEN TAKE-CHARGE STEPS

Positive food swings are the key to an efficient metabolism. They provide essential nutrients, prevent disease, and counter dysfunctional food tendencies. To make positive food swings habitual, follow the seven take-charge steps:

1. Acquire self-determination.
2. Know what to eat.
3. Know how to eat.
4. Establish emotional self-discipline.
5. Know when and what not to eat.
6. Exercise.
7. Take responsibility for stress.

1. Acquire Self-Determination

High-performance primary food swings begin with a commitment to eating well. Getting results in any arena boils down to how badly you want them. The things that matter most in your life—your marriage, your career, your golf game—thrive on commitment and collapse without it. Establishing positive food swings is no different. It requires patience, practice, and occasional failure.

When you refuse to settle for anything but optimal health, you have found the path to primary food swings. The world is filled with sugar-frosted distractions. The challenge is to close your eyes to these temptations and turn your focus inward to your own intentions, so that when you stumble—an inevitable part of any learning process—you won't feel like a victim of external factors beyond your control, but will know, instead, that you have the power to correct yourself. Commitment to self enables you to weather the ups and downs that can discourage other beginners. Your self-determination feeds your commitment.

When learning to take charge of your food swings, a good deal of behavior modification comes into play. You'll also find yourself calling upon your belief systems. If you genuinely believe that it's to your advantage to empower your immune system, prevent degenerative disease, and slow down the aging process with high-performing smart foods, it will be easier for you to stick to it. If, on the other hand, you feel only a vague sense of obligation to eat right "because the doctor said so," your resolve will soon falter.

Make the commitment to high-performance nutrition today. Tell yourself: "I want more out of life!" Believe that you deserve it, and determine to achieve it.

2. Know What to Eat

In the first part, specifically in Chapter 5, I outlined what to eat. Antioxidants got the green light, and anti-nutrients the red light. Naturally, beyond the benefits of high-performance fuel, you will want your diet to be appetizing and emotionally rewarding, so it's important to experiment with a combination of healthy meals to find your preferred menus. Loving your meals will help to keep you motivated.

3. Know How to Eat

Also in the first part, specifically in Chapter 6, I outlined the Golden Rules of Smart Eating. When you are under duress, it will be more difficult, but also more rewarding, to follow these guidelines. In fact, it is at times of stress that you most need the support of smart food swings—to nourish, energize, and calm your nerves. You need a nutritional program that can be counted on to hold up over time and under pressure. The Golden Rules provide a foolproof system, invulnerable to the attacks launched by depression, exhaustion, restaurants, travel, whatever.

It takes time, trial, and error to make balanced undereating a regular habit:

- It takes about twenty-one days to get organized and initiate your meal plan.
- It takes three to four months to establish your new eating habits.
- It takes about two to three years to make the habits permanent.

Two to three years may sound like a long time—until you compare it to your previous life of improper eating.

4. Establish Emotional Self-Discipline

Emotional self-discipline is the yang to the yin of self-determination. Self-determination is largely about mind control. Emotional self-discipline, on the other hand, requires that we succumb to and truly experience our feelings, instead of stifling them with food.

We humans hate to feel vulnerable, and will do almost anything to avoid it. Some of us overeat. Others depend on alcohol, drugs, religious fanaticism, compulsive gambling or sex. Anything to numb the fear. Because we are accustomed to bottling up and blocking out pain, frustration, disappointment, and anxiety, these emotions often trigger negative food swings. We deny our feelings, turn instead to food for a quick-fix mood change, and snack our upsetting emotions into submission.

To change this dysfunctional coping mechanism, we have to summon the courage to face our every feeling and accept that certain days will be better than others. Just like the weather, sometimes it's sunny, sometimes it rains. Each has it benefits, each contributes to the Earth's biological balance. The

same applies to our emotional climate. If we were ecstatically happy every single day, our life would lack nuance and depth, and the potency of all that happiness would be lessened by its prevalence.

Although negative emotions disturb our comfort zone and interfere with our sense of security, they are a part of everyday life. Keep in mind that emotional self-discipline prevents emotional burnout, a state of mind where you have lost full connection to your feelings or moods. Regrettably, most of us have been brought up to regard bad moods not as currents to ride out but tidal waves that might drown us. Instead of dealing with disappointment and frustration, we medicate ourselves with our mommy-daddy diet. But to achieve emotional self-discipline, we need to prepare ourselves for emotional troubles. Emotional self-discipline empowers you to say no. As soon as you recognize that you're feeling upset—but before you reach for the plate of brownies—take alternative action. First, allow yourself to experience your emotions: **Emotional self-awareness is the basis for emotional self-discipline.** Then, after the initial discomfort has passed, start to put the emotions into perspective. Finally, nurture yourself in a way that does not involve a food reward. Put on a favorite CD. Light a scented candle. Phone a close friend. Wrap yourself up in a blanket and read a good book for fifteen minutes. Or take a short walk to appreciate the season, whatever it may be.

Each time you handle emotional tension with positive action, you practice emotional self-discipline. By dealing with your true feelings, good and bad, you are taking responsibility for your emotional life and honoring your emotional needs. You're connected, in touch with yourself.

EMOTIONAL STRENGTH MAKES THE DIFFERENCE

Emotionally repressed individuals have their internal signals mixed. It's tough for them to sort out problems because they're so accustomed to burying everything. They're shut down and burned out, caught in a cycle of oxidative food swings.

Emotionally relaxed individuals, on the other hand, do not use the excuse of food to take the edge off a rotten day. They have the strength to say no to negative food swings, and to choose positive action instead. But this strength is not an innate characteristic. It's earned, ironically, through vulnerability. Emotional self-discipline results when you love yourself enough to tune into, experience, and respect your every emotion. Valuing your feelings is the first step toward establishing a positive belief system, one that can sustain you in the face of adversity.

It deserves repeating: Emotional self-awareness is the basis for emotional self-discipline. When you are emotionally self-aware, you know:

- what you are feeling
- how to experience your feelings, good and bad
- how to evaluate your feelings, and put them in perspective
- how to positively alter your mood and attain your goals

You have the skills necessary to resolve emotional conflict.

FIND YOUR CENTER

In tandem with self-determination, emotional self-discipline prevents negative food swings. Without a clear mind and an open heart, it's easy to use food to relieve tension. Deal with the emotions that drive you to eat and you can reprogram your response to stress.

Recognize, too, that if stress is completely overwhelming you, and has been for a long time, you likely have some self-destructive belief systems in place. Yes, the problem is on the outside, but, more important, it's also on the inside. We can rarely control the outside—the commute, the boss, the in-laws. Our only hope is to adjust the inside. Behaviors you created to protect yourself have become patterns that only repeat the cycle of pain. To break the habit, face the emotions you're avoiding.

Practice these steps toward self-determination and emotional self-discipline:

1. Commit to believing in yourself everyday.
2. Give yourself a chance: Don't beat up on yourself for bad feelings or minor failures.
3. Close your eyes, meditate, focus, and identify how you're feeling.
4. Recruit faith, however you perceive it, to determine what it will take to feel better.
5. Take positive action: Communicate how you feel; connect to yourself and others; nurture yourself without food or drink.

Emotional self-discipline puts you in touch with the bottom of your heart, the depths of your soul. You handle your emotional tension, instead of transferring it to something destructive, such as food. You don't act it out, you work it out.

SMART FOOD CAN COME TO YOUR EMOTIONAL RESCUE

I've already talked about the emotional crutch provided by mommy-daddy diets. The good news is, smart foods can add to your emotional fulfillment, but in a 100 percent healthy way. By keeping you energized, in shape, and disease-free, smart foods help you to feel good about yourself in a way cupcakes never can. The pleasure of a cupcake is fleeting. Ultimately, it boomerangs and backfires. Whole foods, on the other hand, are quiet, steady, constant.

5. Know When and What Not to Eat

Everyday hundreds of physicians send thousands of patients to their local pharmacies to purchase drugs. And everyday millions of Americans add over-the-counter aids to their shopping carts full of prescriptions. But there's one item that cannot be bought or sold: **nutritional common sense**. Nutritional common sense clicks on when you're about to eat something you don't need or even want—probably an item that can be categorized as one of the Top Ten Stress Foods.

As discussed in Chapter 6, abstaining from food is an important principle of prosperous nutrition. Knowing when and what not to eat is skillful, intentional neglect. When nutritional common sense, mental determination, and emotional self-discipline join forces, you'll find the power to say no to fats, sweets, red meat, junk food, and sugary desserts. Nutritional common sense is like the dietary equivalent of your conscience—it's the little voice inside your head telling you that maybe what you're about to eat isn't such a grand idea. It encourages you to avoid unhealthy food swings, just as your judgment encourages you to avoid unhealthy relationships.

In the last chapter, I outlined the Golden Rules for Smart Eating. Those were "the do's." What follows are "the don'ts." When the traffic light is red, you don't drive through the intersection. When the sign says Stop, you don't go. When a school bus brakes, you don't pass it. These are basic rules of the road that you must learn in order to avoid accidents. The same holds true for

eating. Follow the rules, and you'll avoid the nutritional traumas that accompany oxidative food swings.

THE FUNDAMENTAL DON'TS

KEY: DON'T BE A VICTIM OF NERVOUS EATING HABITS!

- DO NOT OVEREAT.
- DO NOT EAT WHEN EMOTIONALLY UPSET, ANXIOUS, OR DEPRESSED.
- DO NOT EAT ANTI-NUTRIENTS OR CHEMICALLY TOXIC FOOD.
- DO NOT SNACK, DOUBLE UP ON SERVINGS, INDULGE IN "JUST A TASTE," OR RAID THE REFRIGERATOR.
- DO NOT BINGE ON CHEESE, CRACKERS, NUTS, FRUITS, OR DRIED FRUITS.
- DO NOT OVERDOSE ON ANY FOOD ITEM FROM ANY FOOD GROUP.
- DO NOT SNACK WHILE YOU ARE COOKING.
- DO NOT EAT DINNER AFTER 8:00 P.M.
- DO NOT EAT WHEN STANDING, DRIVING, OR WORKING.
- DO NOT TAKE YOUR DIET FOR GRANTED.
- DO NOT DRINK WITH YOUR MEALS.
- DO NOT MIX FRUITS AND VEGETABLES IN THE SAME MEAL.
- DO NOT ADHERE TO DIETARY EXTREMISM (TAKE EVERYTHING IN MODERATION).
- DO NOT INDULGE IN CYCLES OF FEASTING AND FASTING.

KEY: JUST SAY NO TO:

- REFINED WHITE SUGARS AND REFINED WHITE CARBOHYDRATES
- SALT
- HYDROGENATED COOKING OILS
- HYDROGENATED NUT BUTTERS
- CANNED, PACKAGED, FROZEN, AND PROCESSED FOODS, OR FOODS WITH TOXIC PRESERVATIVES
- RICH, DAIRY-BASED DESSERTS
- GREASY, FATTY, FRIED FOODS
- HIGH-FAT DAIRY PRODUCTS
- RED MEAT AND OTHER ANIMAL PROTEINS
- COFFEE AND NON-HERBAL TEA

6. Exercise

In addition to burning calories, regular exercise has a beneficial effect on your brain chemistry. It is the most natural anti-depressant. Neuro-endorphins released into the bloodstream increase a sense of well-being and reinforce mind-body balance. Exercise also releases pent-up physical tension, increases energy, and regulates appetite. In short, it's a no-lose proposition.

7. Take Responsibility for Stress

Applying the secret formulas described in Chapter 5 will go a long way toward reducing stress. In addition, when confronted with stress, keep in mind these five general principles:

Know what not to eat. I've said it many times before, but it really does cut to the heart of so many food-related problems. Bad food can do more harm than good food can do well. Anti-nutrients destroy your emotional and physical health. Stay away from high-fat, low-fiber, mucus-forming, acidic foods. Know what not to eat and reduce your stress levels substantially!

Simplify your life. It can be done! First, figure out what really matters to you. Then restructure your lifestyle to honor these priorities. To get started, take this quick test: On a piece of paper, jot down the top three priorities in your life. Next to them, list the three things that take up most of your time. How did the two columns match up? Three for three? When your priorities don't correspond to the way you delegate your time, you need to reevaluate.

If you want to devote more attention to your spiritual growth, do you really need the distraction of seventy-five TV channels? Is that higher salary worth the extra two hours you'll spend in transit everyday? Ask yourself the tough questions. Ask yourself what can go. Then get rid of it. Emotional deprivation is an invariable byproduct of chaos, confusion, and clutter.

Lighten up your life. Most Americans suffer from a serious overload of . . . seriousness. Our culture doesn't value relaxation. But imagine for a moment if you could replace all the stress in your life with relaxation. What a wonderful world it would be! Relaxation requires letting go and lightening up. And it won't impede your professional progress. After all, it's common knowledge that people perform better when they feel calm, secure, and confident, as opposed to irritable, afraid, and impatient. So value downtime in your life. Make it a point to have fun. Encourage your sense of humor. As much as possible, release all the heavy emotional burdens that may have a grip on your heart—face them, express them, grieve, then let go. And strive to shift your attitude toward stress: Consider each predicament an opportunity for growth and self-healing.

Be the captain of your ship. Be the hammer, not the nail; the general, not the foot soldier. See yourself as your own leader, and not as the pawn of a million societal influences outside of your control. This is where your perceptions and beliefs are put to the test: When you feel you are trapped in a dead-end job, loveless marriage, or sickly body, you can consider yourself a victim. But a positive mental attitude and belief in yourself (a) can keep you from ever getting caught in such negative situations to begin with, and (b) if stuck, can help you to manage and eventually transcend your circumstances.

A captain is visionary, opportunistic, strong-willed, goal-oriented. She doesn't sit around waiting for orders. She takes charge! Some might suspect that all that responsibility would add to a stressload. Quite the contrary. When you are in control of your own destiny, when you live by your own personal code, you attain a level of self-respect that greatly reduces stress.

Make Happiness a Habit. Happiness is the cure for stress-related, psychosomatic illness. Determining what makes your heart sing, then going after it with gusto, is the sure path to happiness. Following your dreams sparks the divine within. So love yourself enough to believe that you deserve to be happy, and devote more time to the pursuit of your personal happiness than you currently do to your stress.

CHAPTER 8

APPETITIS: WHAT IT IS
AND HOW TO CURE IT

Life is a prism. What you see depends on what you're looking for. When you feel good and your heart is pure, your life vision sees to it that all your dreams are possible. When you don't feel well and your emotions are shut down, you miss out on the full message of love. When you are ambushed by tension and fatigue, you cannot see positively. Self-abusive food swings only cloud the senses further.

Dysfunctional, or oxidative, food swings dull the emotions and tax the body. Even though common sense alone tells us that poor eating habits turn into harmful food swings, the occurrence of oxidative binges has only increased with the inflationary stress levels of modern-day living. For example, even though the media devotes more attention than ever to nutrition and fitness, the percentage of obese Americans is at an all-time high.

A careful look through the prism reveals that a common affliction unites all the faulty food swings—an affliction I call *appetitis*.

APPETITE VS. HUNGER

Just as tonsillitis is an inflammation of the tonsils and hepatitis is an inflammation of the liver, appetitis refers to an inflammation of your appetite. Let's make a clear distinction between your hunger and your appetite. **Your appetite is your desire for food. It is your emotional hunger. Hunger is your need for food.** When your fuel reserves have been depleted, the resulting physiological state is hunger. A motivational mechanism, hunger encourages you to eat in order to avoid starvation. To express its concern, your stomach growls. Prolonged hunger and a lack of food leads to underconsumption malnutrition. My point being, hunger originates from physical, rather than emotional, need.

Hunger is a state of body. Appetite is a state of mind.

TOO MUCH OF A BAD THING

Many Americans suffer from overconsumption malnutrition—eating too much of the wrong things. This dysfunctional tendency is appetite-driven, influenced by sight, smell, and thought. Everything from social circumstances to sexual innuendo to the sound of burgers grilling on the barbecue can prompt the appetite.

Appetitis is a mood disorder in which emotional needs dictate food choices and the body can hardly recognize genuine hunger any more. Fatigue and food rituals can be underlying causes, but in most cases of appetitis, emotional stress is the culprit. Emotional deprivation leads to unpleasant emotional stress. The emotional tension results in a bad mood. To ease the unpleasant feelings, those in the grip of appetitis reach for food to counter their emotional deprivation.

Emotional Deprivation → Emotional Stress → ↑ EMT → Bad Moods → ↑ EMT → In search of a crutch → Appetitis → Food Swings

EIGHT IS ENOUGH

Acute appetitis can control your emotional life. The mind becomes fixated on crackers and cheese, a box of donuts, a rack of barbecue ribs, and until you answer the craving, it dominates your thinking. The manifestations of chronic appetitis can vary, but eight of the most common dysfunctional food swings are:

1. Overeating
2. Food addiction
3. Compulsive bingeing
4. Snacking and nibbling
5. Food-on-the-brain Syndrome
6. Cravings
7. Late-night indulgences
8. Poor food choices

Appetitis demands aggressive treatment. Because of its cyclical, recurrent nature, it can be difficult to reverse. Natural therapies such as nutritional and emotional detox can be of great benefit.

There is a cure for appetitis: That cure is to stay in touch with your appetite for life. When you are fully connected to your soul, you are too busy living, thinking, and absorbing what is going on around and inside you to be obsessed with your appetite. High-performance foods and my Golden Rules for Smart Eating are also invaluable tools in the quest for appetite control. Both insure that the body is well-nourished at regular intervals, and the balanced chemistry they create helps you to keep a handle on your appetite.

DON'T TRUST YOURSELF

When you are overweight, emotionally stressed, burned out, and off balance, you cannot trust what you think is hunger. You may think you're hungry for a fourth slice of pizza—but you're not. You've already had too much to eat. In fact, you may not have been hungry for the first slice, nevermind the next three. The craving you feel for that candy bar is very real. Unfortunately, it's coming from your mind and your mood—not your stomach. You may think you are "dying" of hunger, when more likely you're dying of fatigue, loneliness, depression, or boredom. A warm cup of peppermint or spearmint tea, combined with a change in your physical environment or a few relaxing yogic postures, can quell most appetitis pangs.

Healthy, balanced people experience hunger—and appetite—all the time. They exert a lot of energy, and require high-performance fuel to maintain their peak level of performance. They earn their meals with hard work and vigorous exercise. When faced with a flare-up of appetitis, they put out the fire, because they're in charge of their emotional life. Over time, they've learned to recognize the signs and symptoms, and they summon up their self-determination and emotional self-discipline to douse the flames and stick to the guidelines. Instead of using food to elevate their mood, they seek other, healthier forms of emotional gratification.

Never lose sight of the eternal truth that your health is a cornerstone to your happiness. It's challenging to live a balanced lifestyle when it seems as if everyone around you is under the spell of stress and The Conspiracy's consumerism. At first, curing appetitis and establishing positive food swings may appear to go against society's grain, and be too radical a departure from the frantic, frenzied norm. But the benefits of high-performance nutrition soon compensate for the initial effort required to make smart eating your personal standard. It's a wise investment.

Which is better: a lifetime of preventing problems, or a lifetime of treating problems? The choice is obvious. But if you're already past the prevention phase, don't despair. As you positively alter your eating habits, and thereby treat your problems, you'll be able to work back to the prevention position.

For now, however, we have to repair the damage and put a stop to the hazardous habits that stand in your way. I'm going to break down the "Eight is Enough" dysfunctional food swings so that you can take a targeted plan of attack. But remember, whatever the food swing, all are characterized by obsessive-compulsiveness, and so must be treated behaviorally.

DYSFUNCTIONAL FOOD SWING #1: OVEREATING

Overeating is the single most common destructive food swing. In fact, it's one of the greatest health hazards facing modern society. My simple definition of overeating is this: eating whatever you don't need, especially when you know you do not want to be eating it. Sounds straightforward enough, but it's a rare individual who does not overeat at least once a day.

Being well-fed is considered a sign of success, prosperity—the good life.

Most parents encourage their kids to eat. Oftentimes, it's a way of silencing and calming children. Grandparents court affection with snacks. And, as we've already discussed in detail, for many of us, food equals love. We down our mommy-daddy diets in a desperate attempt to soothe ourselves.

The malignant end point of overeating is obesity, which, in turn, increases the risk for coronary disease, cancer, diabetes, arthritis, hardening of the organs, and stroke. More than half of all Americans are overweight, and some 10 percent of these individuals are morbidly so, carrying an excess of at least a hundred pounds. In some cases, obesity is caused by glandular conditions and genetic predispositions, but the majority of the time it's due to plain old overconsumption.

The antidote to overeating is undereating.

Undereating high-quality foods at regular intervals is the key to creating healthy, life-sustaining swings.

Emotional overeating is a mood disorder. It is a substitute for love and affection. Its root cause is emotional deprivation. As depression, loneliness, and low self-esteem mount, the overeater turns to food for a mood change. Appetite takes over. Overeating becomes a compulsive, involuntary action. Appetitis is in control.

Sometimes, you just want to eat to your heart's delight. It's your birthday or a special occasion. Of course, I don't condone this type of marathon eating, but it can be looked at as "discretionary indiscretion." Chronic overeating, however, is marked by its regularity—the self-destructive binge-fests that occur on any given Tuesday.

Walking away from food when you still have a bit of an appetite calls for the emotional self-discipline I described in Chapter 7. But it will also give you the impetus to achieve in other areas. After all, feeling stuffed and drowsy after you overeat only inhibits your performance.

TERRY IN THE HANDICAPPED ZONE

Terry was the head cashier for large restaurant in southern California. She liked to think of herself as a pleasant and charming person, but over the past six months she had become increasingly irritable. For the last half of the year, her hand and knees had swollen up, and her joints ached so much that she had to stop working.

"Doctor," she confided, "I feel handicapped. I can't vacuum my house, make the beds . . . and now I'm unable to keep up with my job."

At home, Terry had become quite lazy. She did little more than eat, sleep, and watch TV. Since the onset of her arthritis, her husband had taken over kitchen duty. She ate whatever George served her—and he could be counted on to cook up all his favorites: fried steaks, mashed potatoes, then ice cream and cookies to accompany the night's television viewing. At work, Terry sat at her register most of the day. When she wasn't ringing up sales or supervising employees, she sat at her spot and ate. She had ravenous appetitis, downing everything in sight. At 42, 5'7", and 215 pounds, she was about 80 pounds overweight.

I concluded that Terry's arthritic condition was a result of her obesity. When she came to see me, she was motivated to change. She didn't want to be crippled for the second half of her life. By following the techniques I'll outline in this chapter, she quickly began to make progress. In three months, her joint pain began to diminish. In six months, she'd lost 50 pounds and was back at work. By the end of a year, Terry had lost all her extra weight.

Terry is a perfect example of how overeating can prematurely age the body and cause chronic illness. She discovered that the cure for overeating was undereating.

THE R.R.I.E.A. TECHNIQUE

Overeating is typically the result of an inability to deal effectively with personal frustrations. It's a cry for help. The R.R.I.E.A. technique—which I outline below—answers the call and cures overeating—as well as all the other dysfunctional food swings. I'll be referring to this important technique again throughout the rest of this book, so let me spell out exactly what it is. Make a note of this page, as you may want to refer back to it again.

R: Responsibility

The first step is to take full **responsibility** for your bad eating habits. No one else is to blame. It's easy to come up with excuses: "It was my cousin's wedding," or "I had a hard day" or "I've followed my diet for two weeks, I've earned a break." Remember, the "R" stands for **responsibility**—not rationalization. Commit to curing your own worst habits.

R: Recognition

You've admitted to yourself that you're responsible. Now **recognize** that you are an overeating addict. **Recognize** that you're hooked on the junk. And it's destroying your quality of life. You have no energy. You hate your appearance. You're constantly sick.

Inventory your overeating habits. **Recognize** THAT you overeat, **recognize** WHEN you overeat, **recognize** WHAT you overeat, **recognize** HOW MUCH you overeat. Write it down. Teach yourself to **recognize** your own particular food traps.

I: Identify

Just as you've recognized your food traps, so, too, must you **identify** your emotional state when you are about to, or are in the process of, overeating. To cure the overeating food swing, you have to be connected to yourself. How are you feeling before and during your overeating? Are you really hungry? Ask yourself these two questions every single time you eat, until you know the difference between genuine hunger and deceptive appetitis. Eventually, you'll come to realize that when you are overeating, it's probably because food is available, and that you crave comfort or an emotional reward. Sometimes it can be that someone is expecting you to eat, and you feel obligated.

Identify if you eat to entertain yourself. Is food the main event, the most important part, of your day? Do you eat for fun? Before you begin another eating binge, **identify** the nature of your appetitis with this quick quiz:

- What is overeating doing for me?
- Why do I need to eat at this exact moment?
- What is the benefit of eating too much food?
- What is the benefit of eating unhealthy food?
- What is my predominant emotion—how am I feeling?

E: Express and Experience

The minute you catch yourself overeating, put the food down and **express** your feelings. Say it out loud if that will make it more real. If it involves another person, let her or him know. For example, if you reach for the chocolate-covered pretzels whenever you're frustrated with your kids, next time, as your aggravation escalates, take a deep breath, and calmly say—to yourself, or your children—how upset you are.

Tell it like it is.

If that type of unedited self-**expression** feels too unnatural to risk, then at least start by writing it down in a journal.

The other dimension to the letter "E" is **experience.** You've just said how you feel: Now live it. **Experience** the sad, discouraging, enraging sensations that make you reach for the French fries. When you engage your true emotions, your tension decreases, as does the likelihood that you'll be driven to indulge. Stay with your feelings, even when they're painful. Work through them to a place of inner peace. Meditate. Go deep. Find your center of tranquillity, and notice how the tensions recede.

As you allow yourself to **experience** your emotions, ask:

- What will it take for me to let go of this tension?
- What will it take for me to let go of this preoccupation with food?

You'll likely find that overeating is an escape mechanism, developed to help you avoid harsh emotional realities.

A: Action

Get on the bus, Gus. Make a new plan, Stan. You may not need fifty ways to leave your dysfunctional food swings, but you've got to take meaningful **action.** Substitute a new form of behavior to deal with your emotional distractions. Brew a mug of mint tea. Take a walk. If you're in a restaurant, excuse yourself from the table, then recollect yourself in the restroom. Don't eat. Don't chew gum. Use water, tea, broth, juice, or Re-Vita* as a substitute for biting, chewing, and swallowing. Turn to a loved one for support. Think positive. Repress the hand-to-mouth reflex by doing something else with your fingers—playing the piano, writing a thank-you note, punching a bag.

POSITIVE REINFORCEMENT

The R.R.I.E.A. technique gets results. It is the essence of effective cognitive behavior therapy. The cognitive phase is your becoming aware of your habit. Once you internalize this new reality, you can then take action and
*See Resource

change your behavior. In time, with consistent repetition, it will help you distinguish appetitis from true hunger, cure emotional overeating, and establish constructive food habits. It's all about positive reinforcement—as I said earlier, a behavioral approach.

Here's a summary of the R.R.I.E.A. technique—you may want to photocopy this and stick it on your refrigerator door, or carry it with you and use it as a reminder when you're fighting the appetitis urge.

THE R.R.I.E.A. TECHNIQUE GETS RESULTS!

R: Take **RESPONSIBILITY** for your circumstances.

R: **RECOGNIZE** that you're stuck, and acknowledge that you could be more fulfilled.

I: **IDENTIFY** your negative mental attitude and the limits you place on your expectations. Is your outlook dominated by fear? Is your thinking patterned after your dysfunctional food swings—inconsistent, up and down, constantly fatigued?

E: Honestly **EXPRESS** how you feel about your situation, and allow yourself to **EXPERIENCE** the full range of emotions you've been suppressing.

A: Take **ACTION** and make the necessary adjustments in your attitude and behavior in order to affect positive change.

DYSFUNCTIONAL FOOD SWING #2: FOOD ADDICTION

Overeaters can often be identified by their obesity, but anyone can get caught up in food cravings. One of the great ironies of food addiction is that junk food junkies usually eat food to feel better, but that very food ultimately makes them feel worse. A compulsive quest for a mood change, brought on by taking pleasure in permissive eating, defines the food-addiction food swing.

Food addicts have a lot in common with alcoholics, shopaholics, sexaholics, workaholics, and compulsive gamblers. They eat in spite of themselves and the adverse consequences of their actions. This is the hallmark of classic obsessive-compulsive behavior.

Food obsession is an early symptom of food addiction. If you're always thinking of your next meal, completely preoccupied by thoughts of eating, you're officially obsessed. Eventually, this mind-set manifests itself in an inability to resist the culinary objects of your desire—sweets, salty snacks, starches, breads, and cheese. Food obsession also leads to bingeing.

JANICE THE DONUT JUNKIE

Janice loved glazed donuts. They were the highlight of her day. Yet the whole time she was indulging, she knew it was food insanity—chocolate-covered madness. But she couldn't stop herself, even when she'd start to feel a headache coming on from all the sugar consumption. Instead, she'd continue eating, then take a variety of aspirins, and ride out the pain until it subsided, a few hours later. By evening, when the stress of preparing dinner for her family began to take over, she'd start fantasizing about donuts again.

As an addiction progresses, sneaking food becomes more commonplace. Janice kept an emergency box of donuts hidden in her linen closet, where no one else in the house would ever think to look. Psychologically, this behavior is doubly damaging: Not only is the addict still indulging in the preferred junk items, but now s/he is also deceiving family and friends. Addicts become very uncomfortable when their preferred foods are not available. They begin manipulating people and situations to insure access to their favorite items. Common patterns include:

- Eating "out of sight": in the bathroom, closet, car, backyard, or tool shed
- Eating food secretly, and stashing it in hard-to-find places
- Not eating at parties or out dining with others, only eating at home, later
- Buying food supposedly for your spouse or kids, when you really intend to eat it yourself

Excuses, exclusions, and exemptions mark food addiction. Addicts see food as the perennial pick-me-up, and are prone to blaming their obsession on stressful life circumstances. Food is their main source of security, although, in actuality, their dysfunctional food swings lead to fatigue, irritability, and depression. The clandestine behavior of food addicts—all that sneaking around—adversely impacts their personal relationships, too.

ROXY'S ROAD

Roxy considered herself the life of the party. A friendly, caring, forty-five-year-old, she got a kick out of being the center of attention. And she was accustomed to having a man in her life. But when she met me for her first consultation, she was in the middle of some emotionally traumatic experiences. She had decided to end a seven-year relationship with her lover, Grant. She'd previously been married, but the eighteen-year union ended in divorce. Her only child, Doug, was a senior in high school and living at home. Grant was still married to his second wife, and had three children from his first marriage. Over the course of their relationship, Grant floated back and forth between Roxy and his wife. To me, the situation sounded like an emotional train wreck, but Roxy considered her relationship with Grant the closest thing to true love she'd ever experienced. She and Grant could talk all night long, the sex was great, and he brought out in her a creative side she never knew she had.

Whenever Roxy was with Grant, she felt whole. Whenever he returned to his wife, she was devastated. After seven years of this wrenching pattern, and some intense soul-searching, she finally decided that they had no future. So she gave Grant an ultimatum, and he chose his wife.

Roxy was 5'10" and 210 pounds. She'd gained twenty pounds in the last two months, over the course of ending her affair. She explained her habits to me with exasperation:

"Doctor Meltzer, I am addicted to food. I've tried every diet out there, and I can't take it anymore. I'm tired of playing the social butterfly. In my job as a bookkeeper, I have a lot of deadlines to meet. I'm not big on sweets, but I eat peanut butter and crackers all day long at work. I love rice and potatoes. Sometimes I can't stop eating them."

To counter Roxy's zealous overeating, I prescribed my reliable 600-calorie cleansing diet, and also recommended a daily exercise routine. Her meal plan consisted of:

Breakfast: papaya juice with spirulina or Re-Vita*; ½ cantaloupe
Lunch: leafy green chlorophyll salad with lemon-herbal dressing
Dinner: garden green vegetable salad; 1 cup of steamed green broccoli;
    baked potato, or corn-on-the-cob, or baked squash with salsa—no
    butter or salt on any of them

*See Resource

Within the first week of my cleansing diet, I expected Roxy to lose at least three and up to seven pounds. But when she returned for her second appointment, she'd *gained* seven pounds.

"Roxy," I mused, "on this diet, there is no way in the world you could have gained weight. What happened?"

"Well, Doctor Meltzer," she confessed, "Food has always played a soothing role in my life, and this has been a particularly tough week for me. I've been hungry practically all day long. In fact, I've never felt so low. I have no strength. I tried to follow your diet during the day, but in the evening, when I'm lonely and depressed, I eat. On Tuesday, I 'spaghettied it' all night long. Then I felt too down to go to work the next day. I called in sick, and stayed in bed until noon, with the shades drawn so that I wouldn't know how late it was. When I finally got up, I checked out the fridge. It was filled with fruits and vegetables, so I turned around and went back to bed.

"The phone rang. It was Marta from the escrow company. I'd been planning to move into a new condominium with the money I was going to make from selling my house, but problems came up. The buyer needed more time to meet the down-payment. I'd extended the deadline once already, and I really needed the money now.

"The phone rang again. This time it was Grant. You know how it is when a relationship is in its final stages. We ended up it an ugly argument, I slammed down the phone, and started weeping like a baby. All I wanted was some comfort.

"So I conjured up the idea of spaghetti with onions and cheese sauce. Once I started eating it, I couldn't stop. My son came home from school late in the afternoon, and we decided to make it a pasta party. We ate for the rest of the night. It went on for two days. I didn't get back on your cleansing diet until Friday."

Yikes. Roxy's food addictions were ruining her life, and it took her some time to stick to the R.R.I.E.A. technique. But gradually she began to identify the moods that triggered her binges, address her emotional deficiencies, and take alternative action.

I'm so proud of Roxy, and of the way she taught herself to deal with her frustrations without resorting to food, that I'm going to use her experience as an example of how to employ the R.R.I.E.A. technique. What follows is practically a transcript of how Roxy and I worked through the steps. A caring friend or family member can play my role in the scene. But even if you play both parts, in the privacy of your own kitchen, it is a conversation you must learn to have with yourself. Repeating this technique will improve your abilities to combat food cravings, just as, for example, practicing tennis with better players will improve your game.

THE R.R.I.E.A. TECHNIQUE: "ROXY'S SCENE"

R: Responsibility

Dr. Meltzer: Roxy, in your heart you know that pasta binges are destroying your self-image, depleting your energy, increasing your weight, and putting you at risk for a heart attack. They're ruining your life. Are you prepared to take back control?

Roxy: I'm scared, but ready to be responsible.

Dr. Meltzer: It does require courage, but you have the power within you to change your eating habits.

Roxy: I truly want to tap into that power. I feel like I'm out of touch with it.

Dr. Meltzer: Be patient with yourself. It will take a little time, but if you dedicate yourself to abolishing your dysfunctional food swings, your body will start telling you the difference between appetitis and hunger.

Roxy: Come what may, setbacks and all, I'm committed to the process.

R: Recognition

Dr. Meltzer: In your opinion, what are your food addictions?

Roxy: I recognize that I have a particular weakness for starches and carbohydrates. I find all sorts of creamy, cheesy pastas—ravioli, spaghetti carbonara, manicotti, lasagna—comforting. I also love peanut butter and ice cream. And I have a "salt" tooth: Once I start, I can't stop eating crackers and potato chips.

Dr. Meltzer: Good. Now you know what your refrigerator enemies are.

I: Identify

Dr. Meltzer: Is there a particular time when you feel most vulnerable to bingeing?

Roxy: It pretty much feels like all the time! But it's especially bad when I come home from work and have to face another night alone.

Dr. Meltzer: How are feeling when you are bingeing?

Roxy: Usually, I feel depressed and uptight, tired and lonely.

E: Express And Experience

Dr. Meltzer: Tell me why you feel this way.

Roxy: My seven-year relationship is over—he was married, and the whole thing was one long disaster. I mean, he brought out a lot of my good qualities, but at the same time, the fact that he wouldn't leave his wife was . . . eating away at me. Literally, I guess! And the sale of my house is in limbo, which is completely screwing up my bank accounts. But the tuition for my son's first semester of college is due. And my department at work was downsized, so now I'm doing the job of three people.

Dr. Meltzer: I'm listening.

Roxy: I guess I just feel overwhelmed by all these responsibilities. I feel like I'm drowning. I can't keep on top of the bills, and I'm a total failure at relationships. Sometimes I wonder if I've ever done anything right in my life.

Dr. Meltzer: It must be very painful, but let yourself heal through feeling love for yourself. Unlike physical wounds, which heal with time, emotional wounds do not heal by themselves. It takes work. Work on experiencing your pain by crying, shouting, singing, exercising. Let it out. Write it down. Talk to a trusted friend. Do whatever it takes. Just don't eat.

Roxy: I'm working on it.

A: ACTION

Dr. Meltzer: What's your alternative to indulging in food?

Roxy: I have to catch myself when I'm on the brink of a binge. To blow off steam, I've been jogging. I'll even stop and do ten sit-ups just to regain my focus.

Dr. Meltzer: It also helps to meditate when you feel you're about to lose it emotionally. Find your center, open up your soul, and get in touch with positive vibrations.

Roxy: Sometimes I can do that. It depends where I am, if I can find a peaceful spot.

Dr. Meltzer: Even if you're stuck at your desk at work, summon up a happy memory. And if you're able to truly meditate, end the moment with some creative visualization. Can you do that?

Roxy: Yes. I love to look for pretty shells in the sand, so if I can't actually take get out and go to the beach, then I imagine it. It always makes me feel better.

Play Doctor

Rehearse this exercise until you have mastered the R.R.I.E.A technique. Put yourself in the role of both doctor and patient. Of course, when you play the part of Roxy, add your own dialogue, information that's true to your particular situation. Use the cues as a way to analyze your most recent food fiasco. Relive the experience, your emotions at the time, and visualize how you could have responded differently to your stress. The next time you're confronted with similar circumstances, you'll be better prepared to deal with them constructively.

Be vigilant. Depending on the degree of your food dependency, you may have to go through this self-inquisition five times an hour—some days more, some days less. Stick with it. Pay attention to whatever's missing in your life, and acknowledge that your bingeing is just a form of compensation.

Roxy took up jogging, three miles a day during the week and five on Saturday and Sunday. She became an advocate of the Sunrise Cleanse and Sunset Recharge, meditating twice a day. She changed her habits and her attitude. It took her a few months to wrestle with her demons. Her progress was gradual. But at the end of a year, she had shrunken her stomach and opened her mind. She'd lost 55 pounds and gained control over her emotions. Miraculously, once she accepted herself and her situations, they began to improve. Her escrow finally closed, and she moved into her new condominium. Just as she'd given herself a new look, she made over her home, too. She bought new furniture. And she enrolled in some art classes. In the silence of her meditations, she found that a fear of abandonment was at the root of her food addictions. This revelation made everything clear: Her poor choices in men, her overeating, her anxiety over her housing situation. She was able to put it all in a positive new perspective.

DYSFUNCTIONAL FOOD SWING #3: COMPULSIVE BINGING

Compulsive binging is an extension of food addiction. It's especially common among young women, who may get caught up and trapped in the cycles of binging and purging that characterize bulimia. Although the disorder causes serious damage to the digestive system, and depletes the body of real nutrients, bulimics get hooked on the notion that they can eat as much of whatever they want without gaining weight, because after they've enjoyed the taste of the food, they throw it up. As with other dysfunctional food swings, compulsive binging is dictated by obsessive-compulsive behavior. At first, it allows the addict to feel in charge, but soon s/he becomes a victim of the syndrome, torn between a preoccupation with food and a desperate desire to stay thin. Women in the grips of the condition describe their lives as chaotic. They rationalize that food intake is the only thing they can control, when, in fact, their eating habits are as out of control as everything else.

Vomiting or using diuretics or cathartics only worsens the food addiction. It tricks the body into thinking that it's starving—which, in a way, it is, for true nourishment. The more a binger vomits, the more food the body tries to accommodate the next time around, in a futile attempt to retain nutrients before they are regurgitated.

If you are bulimic, or a compulsive binger, I recommend first that you seek some counseling in order to understand your own specific control issues and the ways in which you apply them to food. Professional support systems are needed to untangle the psychological roots of the disorder; the R.R.I.E.A. technique can be used to change the behavior.

DYSFUNCTIONAL FOOD SWING #4: SNACKING AND NIBBLING

Snacking is about hurried, compulsive eating. Weak and tense nerves like to snack, and snacking damages your nerve endings even further. Snacking can become a crutch and is often seen as an emotional reward system. In fact, snacking and nibbling are so commonplace, we hardly even recognize them as neurotic habits. How could anyone be expected to enjoy the Super Bowl without a buffet full of finger foods? But incessant snacking is a blatant way of releasing nervous energy. The products proliferated by The Conspiracy only enable this syndrome: Almost everything we eat is ready-made—just open the bag or flip the lid, reach in, grab a handful, and pop the prefab food into your mouth. Snacking is the dysfunctional food swing that most exploits the hand-to-mouth reflex and, by extension, what Freud would call our oral fixation. We revert to an infantile stage, and find comfort by replicating an act that reminds us of breast-feeding.

The problem is, we're all supposed to be grown-ups.

Whether it's hors d'oeuvres at a wedding reception or hot dogs at the ballpark, snacking is unavoidable in the average American lifestyle. To begin the process of change, start with moderation: Decide before an event that you will not eat more than x-number of nachos, then stick to your limit. And try to substitute salty snacks with healthier counterparts—fruits and vegetables. As for the dysfunctional extreme of snacking—the compulsive, semi-conscious nibbling that takes place all day long, at home or office, in the car or in front of the TV—well, that's a dead-end food habit. Unless you suffer from diabetes or hypoglycemia and have been prescribed a schedule of snacks that regulates your sugar levels, snacking serves only adverse purposes in your diet.

Compulsive snackers are just as out of touch with their emotions as overeaters and bingers. The difference is, instead of gorging themselves in pig-out sessions, they just nibble, nibble, nibble all day long in order to quiet the anxiety within. But grazing is not good for you. You are not a cow. You are a human being, and constant eating imbalances your metabolism. Snacking confuses your natural hunger mechanisms. Your body never has time to engage the full digestive cycle, because it's always receiving new deliveries into the stomach.

After the initial high of the snack attack subsides, you feel tired. Snacking promotes weight gain: The most common snack foods are high in fat—cookies, potato chips, candy bars, etc.—and snackers overeat these items.

If you are a compulsive snacker, refer back to *Roxy's Scene* on pages 124–126. Put yourself in the role of Roxy, but apply the dialogue to your snacking sickness. The R.R.I.E.A. technique can combat snacking's misguided emotional reward system by helping you to figure out what drives you to indulge and an alternative to this obsessive behavior.

DYSFUNCTIONAL FOOD SWING #5: FOOD-ON-THE-BRAIN SYNDROME

All the dysfunctional swings I've discussed so far—overeating, addiction, binging, and snacking—are characterized by food-on-the-brain syndrome. Those afflicted are fixated by thoughts of shopping for, preparing, and consuming food. They are over-attached to their diets. They use food as an emotional crutch. Life revolves around eating. The only thing that matters is the next meal. They go to bed at night thinking about what they'll eat in the morning. During breakfast, they're planning lunch, at lunch, they're planning dinner. In the middle of other activities, even exercise, their thoughts wander.

Do you spend more time thinking about food than about how to improve your relationship with your spouse, how to be more creative at work, how to accomplish long-term goals? Does your appetitis take precedence over your sex life, your intellectual growth, your emotional stability? The ideal mind-set is one in which, when you eat, you fully enjoy the meal, and when the meal is over, you do not think about food again until the next scheduled meal time.

MORNING, NOON, AND NINA

My patient Nina had an interesting, though not uncommon, strain of food-on-the-brain syndrome. A 40-year-old housewife, she took pride in her highly nutritious eating habits, but complained, "Doctor, I am hungry from the moment I wake up each morning." For breakfast, Nina would combine three fresh fruits in a blender with lecithin, high-protein powder, and wheat germ oil. She was so taken with her craving for her A.M. fruit drink, she consulted a number of physicians to determine the cause of her problem. A series of lab tests put her within normal limits. Her internist was baffled.

I instructed Nina to write down everything she ate for one full week, and to include the time and location of her meals. I also asked her to make note of how hungry she felt each time, what her mood was, and what she was doing. When she returned to my office seven days later, still plagued by her morning hunger, I reviewed her dietary survey. Even though she did have her fruit shake every morning, every evening, between the hours of 9:30 and midnight, she'd snack on cold cuts, cheese sandwiches, or chips and dip.

Nina had food on the brain. She didn't eat because she'd earned meals, and she didn't even delight in her meals. Of course, it's only natural to begin to anticipate food as a designated mealtime draws near, but Nina obsessed about eating all the time. As a result, she ate all the time.

When you eat a large meal right before going to bed, you invariably wake up hungry. Instead of expending the fuel through activities, the rest of your body goes to sleep, leaving the digestive system to work all night to process the food. In the morning, your stomach is empty. Thus begins the cycle. To break it, do not eat after 8:00 P.M.—and the earlier you have to get up in the morning, the earlier your dinnertime should be. Schedule some post-dinner social events to get your mind off food and to keep you from snacking in front of the TV. And exercise whenever possible: I advised Nina to do a half-hour of aerobics every morning, before she reached for her breakfast shake.

Food-on-the-brain syndrome confuses the mind and emotions. I strongly recommend getting involved with your diet and taking an interest in growth-oriented nutrition. But there's a huge difference between a healthy attitude and a hazardous obsession. Nina was dependent on food to give structure and meaning to each day. It was her motivating factor—the fruit shake was the thing that got her out of bed in the morning, just as cheese and cold cuts helped her through her day. A positive relationship with your diet is one in which you are attuned to your true nutritional needs. Nina was using food as an emotional crutch.

As with all dysfunctional food swings, a crucial step in reclaiming control requires making the distinction between hunger and appetite. Appetite is triggered by emotional and mental experiences—complex, ingrained, unconscious associations you may make between, for example, insecurity and a need for the calming taste of chocolate. When you suffer from food-on-the-brain syndrome, appetite dominates.

Nina stuck to the R.R.I.E.A. technique and made a dramatic improvement in her eating habits in three short months. She realized she was unhappy with her life as a housewife, and she began to investigate other ways to deal with her dissatisfactions and emotional deficiencies. The last time I saw her, we realized it had been five years since she'd been at the mercy of her obsessions.

DYSFUNCTIONAL FOOD SWING #6: CRAVINGS

Specific cravings can dominate the mind as much as the more general food-on-the-brain syndrome. The first step on the road to recovery is to realize that **whatever it is you crave, it's almost guaranteed not to be good for you**. It doesn't take a rocket scientist to figure out that buffalo wings are loaded with salt and fat. And ironically, cravings are oftentimes actually allergy-provoking.

Just as there's a difference between hunger and appetitis, and a difference between a healthy attitude and a hazardous obsession toward diet, so, too, is there a difference between food preferences and food cravings. You can prefer certain items over others, but there's a range of flexibility to your choices, and you maintain control. When you crave food, however, the intensity of your appetitis overwhelms everything else, and you cannot rest until you feed the beast within. You have to have that candy bar *right now:* Until you do, you can't think, talk, work, sleep, whatever.

Food cravings are frequently caused by temporary chemical imbalances. For example, a craving for candy usually belies low blood sugar levels or candidiasis. Adrenal burnout, liver stress, and diabetes also spark cravings. But specific emotional imbalances can also be associated with common cravings. Check out the following trigger foods to see if any of these examples sound familiar:

- **Bread:** common for those in need of hugs, physical comfort and emotional support; a food staple that offers emotional security
- **Chocolate:** panacea of the love- and sex-starved; PEA (phenylethylamine), present in chocolate, seems to promote a sense of relaxation and well-being; the effect it produces is similar to the feeling of being in love
- **Crunchy Foods:** an outlet for anger and frustration
- **Salt:** counters feelings of depression by stimulating the system
- **Sweets:** a substitute for affection and a stress-reliever
- **Meat:** more common in men; indicates a lust for power; a classic daddy food, associated with male authority
- **Milk or Cheese:** more common in women, especially those hungry for a deeper emotional connection with mommy; milk, cheese, and ice cream are common crutches during such female hormonal states as PMS, pregnancy, and menopause

One of the tricky characteristics of cravings is **trigger food dysfunction**. In other words, cravings not only satisfy an emotional hunger, but precipitate—or trigger—compulsive overeating and all the other dysfunctional food swings, because once you indulge, you want more. That's why it's so important to use the R.R.I.E.A. technique to recognize your trigger foods and identify the emotions that accompany them. It takes willpower and emotional self-determination, but abstinence is the cure for food cravings.

DYSFUNCTIONAL FOOD SWING #7: LATE-NIGHT INDULGENCES

It's the end of another tough day. You've worked hard, weathered the usual ups and downs. You're tired of the red tape, the rules and regulations, the convoluted bureaucracy of contemporary living. At last, you're home, safe for the night behind locked doors. You can finally let down your guard and indulge.

Some people are completely in control during the day, but then eat from the moment they get home from work until they go to bed. The usual suspects—ice cream, cookies, pizza, beer—are popular with late-night indulgers, who often suffer from boredom or sexual frustration. The late-night indulger rewards him- or herself at the end of the day. Like all other dysfunctional food swings, late-night indulgence is a mood-altering behavior. Applying the R.R.I.E.A. technique will reveal that the late-night eater most likely lacks emotional support and comfort. S/he may carry the burden of responsibility for the rest of the family, be the person everyone else relies on. S/he relies on food.

If you're a late-night food addict, give yourself a break. When you find yourself on the brink of bingeing, take a deep breath and ask yourself, "What's really missing in my life?" Recognize that food is acting as a dysfunctional substitute for other flawed or non-existent relationships.

In terms of the action step of the R.R.I.E.A. technique, creative self-expression is often the key to curing late-night food indulgences. Frequently, people don't want to be bothered putting the effort into an after-work activity. They complain that they're tired, and would rather watch television than, for example, take a writing class in Shakespeare's comedies, or volunteer at the local Y, or study African dance. But creative expression can be so stimulating. It has many benefits—you learn something new, you meet new people, you get away from food, and you show self-respect by treating yourself to something positive. If you're married or in a relationship, a shared interest can bring you and your partner closer. Think about it. You deserve something better to look forward to than food.

DYSFUNCTIONAL FOOD SWING #8: POOR FOOD CHOICES

I include this dysfunctional food swing to remind you of the importance of high-performance nutrition, which I've already described in detail in Part 1. Return to Chapters 5 and 6 for a refresher course in smart foods and the Golden Rules.

Anti-nutrients make you feel heavy—physically and mentally. Junk foods dampen your mood and wrap you up in negative routines, such as the sugar cycle. As I discussed in Chapter 7, prevention is always preferable to treatment. Once you indulge in a food swing, it sets a pattern in motion that becomes much harder to break than if you'd never started. Think of the hamster on the wheel, running to stand still.

Nutritious, antioxidant food enriches body and soul. Stop sabotaging yourself, and get real—with your family, friends, coworkers, and that stranger in the mirror. Move forward with the help of R.R.I.E.A. Transform your dysfunctional food swings into primary nourishing food swings.

CHAPTER 9

HOW TO PREVENT MOOD SWINGS

What do **Abraham Lincoln** and Bill Clinton, Marilyn Monroe and Janis Joplin, Mickey Mantle and Mike Tyson have in common? They've all suffered from de-energizing mood swings. Even the most successful people in the world are sometimes overwhelmed by their emotions.

I do not believe that it is humanly possible to stay in the same mood permanently. Even the worst moods will eventually, inevitably swing back in the other direction. A negative mood swing can:

1. **revert** to a good mood
2. **persist** as is
3. **escalate** into a more negative mind-set

1. A negative mood swing can **revert** to a good mood:

Getting your emotions back on track is a tricky business. Sometimes, you can quickly shake off a sour mood. Sometimes, the bad mood can drag on. Happy, well-adjusted people still get tested by the stress and strain of modern-day living, and minor, short-lived mood swings are common. Depending on the situation, they may even be normal, natural reactions to troublesome events or upsetting news. Tragic occasions require different degrees of grief, depending on the individual. But when it comes to those everyday bad moods, the quicker you bounce back, the better your health—physical and mental.

2. A negative mood swing can **persist** as is:

Low-level depression, pervasive malaise, or an indefinable sadness can linger for hours, sometimes days.

3. A negative mood swing can **escalate** into a more negative mind-set:

Bad moods may extend into deeper depression, heightened anxiety, and extreme irritability. Sometimes, these escalations occur suddenly. You may be in the middle of a normal conversation, but within minutes your temper flares and you lose all composure. Other times, bad moods spread slowly, insidiously taking root until you're trapped, and you can't remember when you last felt happy.

A **sudden-onset mood swing** describes the emotional state when a cluster of moods appears on the horizon, then disappears just as quickly, within an hour or two. Sometimes, these swings can be so severe, they occur one after another. This is a symptom of extreme emotional instability, and may indicate borderline manic-depression. It demands the attention of a psychiatrist.

THE EMERGING FIELD OF EMOTO-NUTRITION

In the previous chapter, I discussed my R.R.I.E.A. technique for combating dysfunctional food swings. The objective of this chapter is to explain the intimate connection between moods and eating habits. There are entire new fields of nutrition emerging, fields that deal with such psychosomatic associations. Emoto-nutrition analyzes the dynamic interplay between diet and emotions. The study is founded on two fundamental principles that have evolved over the past quarter-century from the related subject of orthomolecular nutrition, which focuses on the relationship between food and the mind.

We know that our mood is our frame of mind. It is the present state of our feelings. We also know that moods have an enormous influence over behavior, habits, and actions. The first principle of emoto-nutrition is very simple. In fact, you're already familiar with it. It is a recurrent theme of *Food Swings*.

Principle 1: Your Moods Influence Your Eating Habits

We've already established that moods have everything to do with appetite and eating habits. We've also discussed the negative impact poor food choices have on emotional states. Perhaps most important, we've discovered that chronic dysfunctional food swings mask mood disorders and are driven by unresolved emotional tension. The first principle of emoto-nutrition takes these ideas two step further. To begin with, it states that **emotional balance, continued through primary nutritious food swings, leads to nutritional balance, which prevents dysfunctional food swings.**

The corollary to this principle is that emotional balance feeds nutritional balance.

A balanced emotional life is conducive to wholesome, health-enriching eating habits. For your body to thrive, your emotions have to thrive, too. When you are emotionally adjusted, you have the inner strength necessary to stick to high-performance nutrition, even in the face of surprises or disappointments. Emotional balance enables you to effectively manage stress—**and to separate stress from your eating habits**. Your emotional issues and your diet are independent of each other.

Conversely, **emotional imbalance leads to negative mood swings that provoke dysfunctional food swings, which result in nutritional imbalances and, eventually, disease**.

The corollary to this is that emotional imbalance feeds nutritional imbalance.

Principle 2: Your Eating Habits Influence Your Moods

This is the flip side of the equation. **Primary nutritious food swings lead to nutritional balance, which promotes emotional balance, which, in turn, prevents negative mood swings**.

In effect, nutritional balance feeds emotional balance.

Feed Your Mind

High-performance nutrition and primary positive food swings do an excellent job of not only balancing your body chemistry but also

balancing your brain, or emotional, chemistry. They have a steadying, neuro-chemical effect on your emotions.

Food plays a dominant role in determining mood. Primary nutritious food swings empower you to regulate your own neuro-chemical and neuro-glandular systems: your hormones, master glands, neurotransmitters, and nervous system. High-performance food promotes a high-performance liver, pancreas, adrenals, pituitary, thyroid, hypothalamus, limbic system, and immune system. You benefit from a strong set of nerves and a stockpile of emotional strength. You are in a position to take charge of your emotional life and deal strategically with day-to-day ups and downs. And positive food swings are "progenerative"—your body becomes more and more healthy over time, enabling you to quickly adjust to setbacks beyond your control—a virus, for example, or a strained muscle. This ability to maintain your balance is another key to preventing mood swings.

Feed your brain and nervous system smart food and you'll achieve emotional balance. This is the purpose of emoto-nutrition.

As explained above, Principle 1 is a two-way street: Emotional balance feeds nutritional balance, and emotional imbalance feeds nutritional imbalance. In Principle 2, just as nutritional balance feeds emotional balance, so, too, does nutritional imbalance feed emotional imbalance. Poor nutrition and dysfunctional food swings have a negative neuro-chemical influence on your emotions.

THE NEURO-CHEMICAL CAUSE OF MOOD SWINGS

Mood swings are based on an underlying chemical imbalance that alters your brain chemistry. But when you eat smart food, your nervous and glandular systems receive proper nutrients that balance them. Your emotional state is a result of the interaction between your nerves, your hormones, and your psychological profile. The glandular system regulates hormones. The nervous system can either contribute to or detract from hormonal balance. Wholesome food, hormonal balance, healthy nerves—they all go together.

Blood sugar is the primary fuel for the brain. All brain functions, from thinking to willpower to discrimination to mood, depend on a steady supply of this fuel. With high-performance nutrition, nerves and hormones hook up healthily. Metabolic pathways work all day long to convert blood sugar, or glucose, into brainpower and balanced emotions. Within the blood/brain interactions, such hormones as norepinephrine, serotonin, thyroxine, cortisol, and dopamine affect mood. For example, a high serotonin level results in a good mood—this is the main thrust of anti-depressant therapy.

Altered emotional states—mood swings—can often be traced to hormonal imbalances. The nerves and hormones are out of synch. In turn, hormonal imbalances can often be traced to improper eating habits and faulty food selections, which derail metabolic systems—the interrelated workings of glands, hormones, and neurotransmitters. Toxic anti-nutrients get trapped in the nerve endings, then cross the blood/brain barrier as neurotoxins. These neurotoxic anti-nutrients damage brain metabolism. What starts out as an innocent food indulgence for the sake of pleasure ends up causing hormonal imbalances that dampen moods.

PMS and Male Menopause

Individuals who suffer from acute, intense mood swings feel out of control. Their disruptive swings seem to appear without warning. At any given moment, tempers erupt or tears flow. Prevalent mood swings include: panic attacks, temper tantrums, crying fits, sexual frigidity, pensive depression, and mute reclusiveness. They diminish performance at work and in the bedroom. They drain energy, deflate confidence, encourage insecurities, impair judgment, and invite overreaction.

Mood swings affect both sexes. In the days before and during their menstrual period, many women experience a range of emotions, from irritability to sudden sadness. In the past, traditional medicine has discredited PMS, but it's a very real and chronic condition that can be alleviated with the right food choices. For example, vegetables such as romaine lettuce and proteins such as tofu eaten every couple of hours can regulate blood sugar and eliminate cravings.

Many women need to learn to overcome the sexist belief that their emotional life is bigger than they are. As for men, although few would admit it, many slip into a subclinical depression between the ages of 45 and 55. This is what I call the male menopause. Although the midlife crisis has become something of a bad joke, it, too, is affected by concrete neuro-chemical factors. Men have to realize that they are disconnected from their emotional life. This disconnection leads to dysfunctional food swings.

Emotional stability is a sign of good health. But mood swings build emotional tension and bring nervous energy into the body. If you're tired—literally and figuratively—of weathering your weekly moods swings, if you're sick—literally and figuratively—of being a victim of your cravings, if you hunger—literally and figuratively—for emotional consistency, you're ready to eat right. Eating right will balance your brain chemistry and immunize you against mood swings.

THE BLAME GAME

Busy people blame their bad moods on rushing. Frenzied mothers find fault with their neverending chores. Working professionals point to industrial-strength stress and pressures from their boss. Many successful folk leading supposedly fulfilling lives still fall victim to mysterious mood swings that seem to come and go for no apparent reason. What can be done?

Consider the case of Jennifer. She almost always tires in the middle of the afternoon. She has a difficult job, rushes to pick up her daughter from daycare at 5:30, and struggles to get dinner on the table by the time her husband gets home, close to 7:00. When she feels down, Jennifer reaches for cookies, but within an hour and a half, she's more tired and irritable than before. Her fatigue persists until she gets a good night's sleep, but then she goes through the same swings the next day.

BE ON THE LOOKOUT FOR LOW BLOOD SUGAR

Some erratically moody individuals suffer from underlying personality disorders, but most are simply stuck in a cycle of stress-related food swings. As illustrated in the wheel on page 98, hormonal imbalances cause mood swings. Now here's the clincher, the last piece in the puzzle: The great majority of the time—I'd put the number at around 85 percent—fluctuations in blood sugar cause the imbalances that trigger mood swings.

Yes, functional hypoglycemia is the most common cause of de-energizing mood swings. Other nutritional and/or metabolic imbalances can also bring on mood swings, but low blood sugar is by far the most likely culprit. In fact, I'll even go so far as to say that mood swings are synonymous with the symptoms of fluctuating blood sugar. Lactic acid buildup, liver malfunctions, suppressed immune systems, and undiagnosed food allergies round out the top five causes of mood swings. Interestingly, these other four conditions are also complications of faulty food swings. All five are associated with abnormalities in carbohydrate metabolism.

THE TOP FIVE CAUSES OF MOOD SWINGS

1. LOW BLOOD SUGAR
2. LACTIC ACID BUILDUP (OR LIAS, LACTATE-INDUCED ANXIETY SYNDROME)
3. LIVER DYSFUNCTIONS
4. COMPROMISED IMMUNE SYSTEM
5. FOOD INTOLERANCE OR UNDIAGNOSED FOOD ALLERGIES

1. Low Blood Sugar

Mood swings are a classic symptom of burnout: Low blood sugar is the chemistry of burnout. Oscillations in blood sugar, in thirty-minute intervals a few hours after eating, characterize reactive or functional hypoglycemia. Glucose levels drop and peak, again and again. The rate, duration, and intensity of the drops determines their impact.

With the help of healthy food swings, the body can maintain its blood sugar within a sensible range before, during, and after you eat. In a balanced metabolism, blood sugar doesn't climb too high (diabetes) or drop too low (functional hypoglycemia). This state of equilibrium is the result of teamwork between the liver-pancreatic-adrenal axis and the pituitary-thyroid-adrenal axis—two collectives of organs and glands that regulate glucose and hormone levels. But if the control mechanisms are overloaded or burnt out, blood sugar irregularities result.

The pancreas secretes insulin and glucagon. Insulin lowers blood sugar levels; glucagon raises them. The two hormones work together to stabilize blood sugar and supply energy. Insulin enhances the body's utilization of glucose as cellular fuel, and facilitates its uptake into muscles and other tissues. When blood sugar gets too low, glucagon sends a message to the liver to release some glycogen, for a boost.

The adrenals serve as a backup system to the pancreas's regulating mechanism. When blood sugar rapidly declines, or when you are jolted by fear, the glands release adrenaline (epinephrine) and other steroids. These adrenal hormones work to break down stored glucose and elevate blood sugar, so that more energy is available when needed. But a problem arises when high levels of oxidative stress cause the pituitary-thyroid-adrenal axis to wear down and burn out. Without fully functioning adrenals, the body lacks the energy to access stored glucose and increase blood sugar levels.

Adrenal burnout leads to low blood sugar.

The combination of poor diet and oxidative stress—with its negative impact on the adrenals, pituitary, thyroid, liver, pancreas, and nervous system—sets in motion a cycle of hypoglycemic food swings.

Remember that glucose fuels the brain, just as it fuels all other organs. When blood sugar drops, the brain and nervous system are the first to be adversely affected. Common symptoms include anxiety, depression, fatigue, irritability, mood swings, nervousness, and craving for sweets. Sweating, shaking, headaches, blurred vision, and dizziness—especially upon standing up—may also occur. When any of these symptoms appear within a few hours of eating, functional hypoglycemia must be ruled out as the culprit.

Refined White Sugar and Carbohydrates Cause Low Blood Sugar

Medical experts generally agree that overconsumption of white refined sugars and carbohydrates debilitates the body's glucose control mechanisms by causing stress to the liver-pancreatic-adrenal axis. A diet high in white refined carbs and sugars—found in cookies, cakes, soft drinks, and dried, sweetened fruits—results in functional hypoglycemia. In spite of this, most Americans derive nearly one-third of their daily calories from refined sugars and sugars added to processed foods as sweeteners. A 1989 study by the National Research Council ("Diet and Health Implications for Reducing Chronic Disease Risk"; Washington, DC, National Academy Press) concluded that the typical individual consumes more than 100 pounds of sucrose and 35 pounds of corn syrup every year.

Clinical nutritionists also concur that low blood sugar causes foggy brain functioning. Think of it this way: The brain is dependent on glucose just as the lungs are dependent on oxygen. When the ratio of either is askew, your body will feel off-balance. Decreased mental capacity—the inability to concentrate or to remember, for example—is an early warning sign of low blood sugar. It usually precedes a mood swing. Treat functional hypoglycemia in its early stages, before it critically affects the pituitary-thyroid-adrenal axis, and you can sidestep a dysfunctional food swing.

By the way, low blood sugar doesn't only dull your thinking. It influences your actions, attitude, and emotions as well. The same National Council study showed that aggressive criminal behavior, even seizures, have been linked to functional hypoglycemia.

The High Fiber, Complex Carb, Complete Protein, No Sugar Plan

Functional hypoglycemia can be cured. To stabilize blood sugar, the most crucial step is to eliminate sucrose and refined carbohydrates from your diet. Then it's all in the timing: Hypogylcemia is a dysrhythmic disorder. To regain control and recalibrate blood sugar levels, it's necessary to eat smaller meals every two-and-a-half to three hours throughout the day, over the course of about three months. Follow these guidelines:

- Eat complex carbohydrates and complete protein at every meal
- Do not eat ANY sweets—not even fruit—for the first six weeks
- Focus on high fiber
- Take pantothenic acid
- Take chromium
- Learn to love licorice
- Avoid alcohol

■ Eat Complex Carbohydrates and Complete Protein at Every Meal

Between meals, snack on complete proteins and some kind of complex carbohydrates (for examples, refer back to Chapter 5). Never let more than three hours pass without eating some protein. A typical day might include:

breakfast: whole grain cereal with nuts
snack: almond butter on seven-grain toast
lunch: avocado or hommus sandwich
snack: rice cakes with almond butter
dinner: whole grain pasta with veggie burger and green salad

The idea is to eat complex carbs and high-fiber foods, with an emphasis on bean and legume protein.

▓ Do Not Eat ANY Sweets—Not Even Fruit—For The First Six Weeks

Absolutely no sweets—candy, cookies, cake, chocolate, ice cream, donuts—and no refined white carbs. No fruit, fresh or dried, for the initial six weeks. The first category, obviously, is sky-high in overprocessed anti-nutrients. The second, although a healthier option in the long-run, still contains natural sugars. In order to rebalance glucose levels, we first have to clean out the system.

▓ Focus on High Fiber

Water-soluble fiber slows down the rate of absorption of complex carbohydrates and proteins. This helps to prevent the rapid rise in blood sugar that often precedes the hypoglycemic drop—the classic up-and-down pattern that sets off a dysfunctional swing. Optimal water-soluble fibers include: almonds, green vegetables, legumes, oat bran, sunflower seeds, and psyllium seed husks.

▓ Take Pantothenic Acid

Pantothenic acid, commonly known as vitamin B_5, builds up the adrenals and leads to better blood glucose control. Take 500 milligrams twice a day (for a total of 1,000 mg daily) for up to three to six months after the symptoms of functional hypoglycemia disappear. The vitamin can be purchased in tablet form at pharmacies or, preferably, health food stores (the drugstore brands are often synthetic and of a lesser biologic potency).

▓ Take Chromium

In the medical profession, chromium is referred to as "the glucose tolerance factor." It helps insulin to process glucose. Supplement your diet with 200 micrograms twice a day (for a total of 400 mcg daily). Like pantothenic acid, chromium is available in pill form at pharmacies and health food stores. It should be taken for six to twelve months.

▓ Learn to Love Licorice

Licorice contains glycyrrhizin, a glycoside. This active herbalite is similar in structure and activity to adrenal steroids. It works to keep blood sugar elevated.

▓ Avoid Alcohol

Alcohol lowers blood sugar by interfering with the body's glucose-regulating mechanisms and causing an increase in the release of insulin by the pancreas.

Alcohol-induced reactive hypoglycemia often triggers cravings for sweets, caffeine, or more alcohol. Thus begins the sugar cycle and its subsequent mood swings.

To understand how refined carbs deregulate the body's glucose levels, it's necessary to understand their composition. In essence, the entire trace mineral content and most of the B vitamins have been extracted from: refined white sugar; refined carbohydrates such as white bread; pastries; and packaged cereals. Because these items are already so highly refined, the digestive system is left with few nutrients to process, and instead the sugars and carbs are rapidly absorbed into the bloodstream. The pancreas reacts to this influx of sugar by releasing insulin, which lowers glucose levels, resulting in reactive hypoglycemia and all its mood-swing, food-swing symptoms. Stabilized blood sugar eliminates most swings.

2. Lias: Lactate-Induced Anxiety Syndrome

A few years ago, hardly anyone had heard the term "lactose intolerant," and even today, people consider it primarily a digestive dysfunction. But lactic acid can also induce anxiety and other mood swings. LIAS, or Lactate-Induced Anxiety Syndrome, describes this condition, a result of lactic-acid buildup in the bloodstream. Symptoms include apprehension, confusion, fatigue, fear, irritability, and other mood changes.

Lactic acid is normally present in the blood during periods of increased physical activity or muscle exertion. Exercise can cause LIAS, but carbohydrates are also often the culprit. Observe the process:

1. In the liver, sucrose, fructose, and refined carbohydrates are converted into glucose.
2. Glucose is then converted into pyruvic acid.
3. Pyruvic acid, in turn, is transformed into energy.

But when there is a deficiency in B vitamins, then pyruvic acid is converted into lactate. Because most of the B vitamins have been removed from refined white sugar and carbohydrates, consumption of these items upsets the pyruvate-to-lactate ratio and increases the amount of lactic acid in the bloodstream. These elevated levels of lactate lead to anxiety.

When you exercise vigorously without breathing properly, or in a stuffy, poorly ventilated environment, and the muscles can't access enough oxygen to burn glucose, then the body reacts anaerobically and lactate builds up. In lactate-sensitive individuals, this can cause panic attacks.

To treat LIAS:

- Follow the high fiber, complex carb, complete protein, no-sugar plan outlined above, for functional hypoglycemia
- Remember to snack between meals on high-protein foods like almond butter
- Do not eat ANY fruit sugar or fructose
- Eliminate caffeine
- Eliminate alcohol
- Reduce anxiety with kava kava
- Take vitamin B_1, 500–1000 mg daily
- Take vitamin B_2, 400–600 mg daily
- Take a calcium supplement, preferably calcium citrate, 1000 mg daily
- Take a magnesium supplement, preferably magnesium citrate or aspartate, 500 mg daily

And in addition to all of the above, take frequent saunas. Sweating profusely is an excellent way for the body to detoxify itself and rid the blood of built-up lactate.

3. Liver Dysfunctions

The liver is directly involved in the glucose process. It stores glucose in the form of glycogen, and when blood sugar drops, the liver goes to work to raise levels back up. It also responds to the prompts of adrenal hormones, and reconverts lactic acid into pyruvate. Obviously, it plays a crucial, constant role in the body's absorption of nutrients and removal of waste. But when the liver's enzymatic systems are damaged by alcohol, drugs, and stress brought on by poor food selections, then excess levels of lactate remain in the bloodstream. To truly detox the liver, in addition to abstaining from refined white sugars and carbohydrates, it's necessary to avoid alcohol, caffeine, dairy products, chicken, seafood, and red meat. A vegan diet can regenerate the liver. Milk thistle can be used to protect your liver function.

4. Compromised Immune System

The immune system protects the body against infection and fights off illness. But when the immune system has been worn out, compromised, or suppressed, even a minimal amount of oxidative stress can provoke a mood swing. The yeast fungus is one of the most prevalent invaders of a weakened immune system. It creates a condition called candidiasis. Because of its effect on the liver and digestive organs, it can cause functional hypoglycemia. It can also cause brain allergies.

Candida, the yeast that causes candidiasis, already lives in the body. When your systems are in balance, you will not know it exists. But once the immune system is weakened, by anything from antibiotic abuse to chronic fatigue to cancer, such physical symptoms as abdominal bloating, constipation, cramping, cystitis, diarrhea, distention, and skin rashes can occur. Emotional symptoms include anxiety, depression, and drastic mood swings.

When candida gets a foothold in the digestive system, it breaks down the normal boundaries between the bloodstream and the intestines, causing bowel problems. Toxins from undigested protein can enter the blood through the intestinal tract, attack the brain as neurotoxins, and consequently cause mood swings by undermining mental functions.

A yeast-free, anti-hypoglycemic diet treats candidiasis. In addition to the strict exclusion of sweets, fruits, refined sugars and carbohydrates, the plan also prohibits dairy products and fermented foods such as vinegar. Any items high in yeast or mold—many breads and cheeses, mushrooms, peanuts, and alcohol, for example—must be avoided at all costs. To kill off excess yeast, it's often necessary to use capryllin or nystatin. Capryllin, or capryllic acid, is a naturally occuring fatty acid that can be taken as an enteric-coated time-released supplement in tablet form, 1000 to 2000 mg with each meal. Nystatin is by prescription only. It's best to start with the anti-fungal capryllin first and then turn to nystatin if it does not work. A patient should not use both at the same time.

A probiotic, to protect the bowel flora, is also helpful. *Lactobacillus acidophilus* or *Lactobacillus bifidum* can help restore healthy intestinal flora. To recolonize the intestinal tract, probiotic supplementation at a dosage of one- to ten-billion cells daily, in liquid or tablet form, for at least six to ten weeks, is advised. I also recommend pancreatic digestive enzymes, taken in tablet form. With the exception of nystatin, all are available over the counter at pharmacies and health food stores.

5. Food Intolerance

If you consistently experience unfavorable reactions to certain foods, it's possible that you're allergic to or intolerant of those items. Food allergies manifest themselves in a number of common immune disorders: chronic ear infections, recurrent bronchitis, acute digestive dysfunctions, lupus and other autoimmune disorders, persistent skin problems, arthritis, and various forms of colitis. Of course, all of these diseases have a negative impact on your mood, but I would argue that not only the consequent sicknesses, but also the causative food, is responsible for anxiety, depression, and turbulent emotions. Food allergies most certainly can affect mental functioning. For example, have you ever experienced strange dreams the same night you've eaten an extremely spicy meal?

When food is not completely digested, fermentation and dysbiosis occur. In other words, partially digested proteins and carbohydrates are stuck inside your body, rotting like leftovers in the fridge. Frightening thought, isn't it? The resulting toxins—the "internal mold," if you will—can cause adverse reactions in the digestive and musculoskeletal systems, liver stress, and can affect the skin. Neurotoxins can damage the central nervous system. In this way, food intolerance or allergy can cause impaired function of your nerves and contribute to dysfunction of your emotions and mood swings.

Most people think of food allergies as instantaneously life-threatening: "If Sally eats strawberries, she'll die." But food allergies can be more insidious. In fact, I'd go so far as to say that functional hypoglycemia is the result of the body's intolerance of sweets and refined carbohydrates. That sugar cookie may not kill you on the spot, but in the long run, it's damaging your systems.

The obvious cure for an allergy is to eliminate the offending food. Sometimes, it's easy to pinpoint the cause of your digestive woes. But often it's necessary to undergo a complete dietary analysis to identify the culprits. For our purposes, I simply want you to be aware that a food allergy or intolerance may be contributing to your mood swings. If you suspect this is the case, investigate further with the help of a nutritionist.

But it's most important to understand that the above five metabolic disorders, from low blood sugar to food allergies, can all be treated without conventional drug therapy. In my experience as a nutritionist, smart foods and a proper diet—plus an honest emotional life—have a strong 85 percent success rate. High-performance food swings prevent mood swings. If you feel you are not responding to the nutritional and emotional healing techniques I've outlined so far, consult a nutritionist, but evaluate your condition with a psychiatrist, too. A nutritionist will analyze the impact of your dietary choice, and a psychiatrist can put them into neuro-chemical perspective.

CHAPTER 10

PHYTO POWER:
THE TEN MOST ENERGIZING FOODS

Conventional dietetics calculates calories as a measure of the amount of energy a particular food item can provide. But calories are a most misleading index. Even though butter, for example, is very high in calories, eating a lot of it will not energize the body. It will, on the contrary, have exactly the opposite effect. Contrary to traditional medical texts or past nutrition classics, more calories do not equal more energy. Why? Because not all food offers the same bounce per ounce.

THE POWER OF PHYTONUTRIENTS

The source of food's power lies not in its caloric quantity but its **phytonutritive** quality. *Phyto* is derived from the Greek prefix which means "from the plant." *Phytonutrient* refers specifically to the energizing enzymes found in fruits and vegetables. Phytonutrients bring the body to life, pepping up nerves, stimulating master glands, invigorating organs and tissues, and recharging brain batteries.

In the past few years, research has indicated that animals fed broccoli and other members of the cabbage family (known collectively as cruciferous vegetables) had lower rates of cancer than those in the control group. Applying the same theory to humans, German scientists discovered that, compared to Americans on the SAD diet, the Japanese suffer significantly lower rates of cancer. The experiments determined that the Japanese had a large percentage of *genistein*—a phytonutrient derived from soy—in their urine. A separate study, based in Italy, revealed that a diet high in tomatoes helped to prevent many digestive cancers. Tomatoes are rich in the phytonutrient *lycopene*. Research at Harvard Medical School involving 50,000 men confirmed that those who increased their intake of tomato-based lycopene reduced their risk of prostate cancer by about 25 percent.

In fact, scientists have recently isolated more than 500 phytonutrients in just one tomato!

Having confirmed the benefits of phytonutrients, scientists specializing in the field are now focusing on the health-promoting compounds within whole foods. They refer to these as **phytochemicals**—the natural chemicals present in the plant kingdom. Thousands can be found in fruits, vegetables, grains, and legumes. Phytochemicals are the biologically active substances that give plants their unique flavors, colors, and therapeutic value. They protect plants against their own plant diseases and, by extension, prevent illness in humans, too.

Phytochemicals bestow medicinal properties upon natural foods. Fruits, vegetables, and whole grains rich in phytochemicals reduce the risk of heart disease, stroke, premature aging, macular degeneration, and most cancers. Potent antioxidants, they protect tissues and cells from potential damage by neutralizing free radicals—the toxic oxygen molecules that cause degeneration and are thought to play a role in the development of cancer. Phytochemicals can also reduce restrictive coronary artery disease. They've been found to block the oxidation of LDL cholesterol, preventing it from turning into artery-clogging plaque. I'm confident there are yet-to-be-discovered phytochemicals that regulate our metabolism and balance our hormones, and still others that stimulate the release of neurotransmitters responsible for our emotional well-being. Some phytochemicals may even protect our DNA from breaking down.

The point being, there is an expanding body of evidence supporting the belief that phytochemicals contain antioxidant, anti-inflammatory, and anti-cancerous properties. And I'm ready to make the next logical leap in reasoning by asserting that phytochemicals in living foods swing the body into a high-energy state. They prevent and heal illness. It's only a question of time until the specific phytochemicals that enhance our emotional well-being are discovered, just as the specific phytochemicals that protect the immune system are now being identified by scientists all over the world.

Choose phytonutritive quality over caloric quantity! The top Ten energy-increasing foods I'm about to list all contain high percentages of phytonutrients. They put a spring in your step. They fill you with *joie de vivre*—passion for life. I consider foods rich in phytonutrients to be the *real* soul food: They help sustain emotional balance, and by enabling you to experience the magnificence of being fully alive, they nurture the spirit as well.

THE TEN MOST ENERGIZING FOODS

1. SPIRULINA AND SUPER-GREEN FOODS
2. CITRUS FRUITS: ORANGES, GRAPEFRUITS, PINEAPPLES
3. BROCCOLI AND OTHER CRUCIFEROUS VEGETABLES
4. ROYAL JELLY
5. BAKED POTATO
6. REISHI AND SHIITAKE MUSHROOMS
7. FRUIT SMOOTHIES
8. SEVEN-GRAIN BREAD
9. VEGGIE BURGERS
10. TEMPEH

1. Spirulina and Super-Green Foods

Spirulina, a blue-green microscopic algae, is one of nature's most potent proteins. Like chlorella, spirulina is referred to as a "super-green" because of its high chlorophyll content. Chlorophyll's molecular structure closely resembles that of hemoglobin, the oxygen-carrying protein found in red blood cells.

Wheat grass and its juice are also high in chlorophyll. Dr. Ann Wigmore, the renowned nutritionist and naturopath, popularized the use of wheat grass to rejuvenate the immune system and treat cancer. Rich in enzymes, bioflavonoids, and vitamin C, it boosts the immune system.

Super-greens are super-alkaline. In addition to energizing the body with their concentration of proteins, minerals, antioxidants, vitamins, and enzymes, they protect against arthritis and other acid-forming conditions.

Note: The harvesting process is critical to the quality of spirulina. Optimally, in the extraction procedure, the temperature does not exceed 88 degrees. For this reasons, I recommend Revita, the Liqua Health version of spirulina (*see Resources*).

2. Citrus Fruits

Oranges, pineapples, grapefruits (particularly pink ones), mangos, and tangerines are all high in enzymes. Their unique chemistry cleanses the blood and breaks up mucus in the lymph system—crucial, because a clogged lymph system decreases energy levels. Citrus also purifies the liver, spleen, and bone marrow. Citrus pulp is rich in anti-allergenic, anti-inflammatory phytonutrients. Citrus juice is high in vitamin C, trace minerals, and electrolytes.

Make citrus fruits a part or your daily nutritional program, especially during the winter months. A freshly squeezed glass of orange, grapefruit, or pineapple juice will give you a healthy boost.

3. Broccoli

Broccoli, a high-chlorophyll cruciferous vegetable, is nutrient-dense and rich in enzymes. It contains a full complement of antioxidants, bioflavonoids, carotenoids, selenium, vitamin E, vitamins B, and phytonutrients. It's especially good for bolstering the immune system—more than any other food, it builds resistance to infection and cancer. It's also high in fiber. Add raw broccoli to a garden salad or mix it with pasta, tofu, or vegetable soup.

Other cruciferous vegetables include cabbage, kale, Brussels sprouts, broccoli rabe, bok choy, cauliflower, mustard greens, and turnip greens. All of these contain the phytonutrient sulphoraphane, as well as other isocyanothianates which stimulate the liver to secrete enzymes that detoxify and dispose of carcinogenic metabolites. Cruciferous vegetables also have indoles, which can inactivate potentially damaging estrogens, and quercetin, which energizes the liver and spleen.

4. Royal Jelly

Royal jelly is a miracle food brought to us by bees. Specifically, it is secreted from the throat glands of nurse bees between the sixth and twelfth day of their life. A combination of honey and pollen gives the substance a thick, creamy texture. Royal jelly is rich in B vitamins, and contains high proportions of two crucial elements: pantothenic acid (vitamin B_5) and acetylcholine. Pantothenic acid nourishes the adrenal glands, where, of course, energizing adrenaline is produced. Acetylcholine, an elemental neurotransmitter, allows nerves to send messages to each other.

Royal jelly's many minerals, hormones, enzymes, and amino acids (it has eighteen) aid the immune system. Try some between meals, when you need a pick-me-up. Royal jelly is commonly available in liquid form, combined with ginseng in vials of 300–500 mg.

5. Baked Potato

The potato deserves its reputation as an energy-boosting staple food. A complex carbohydrate, it helps to build endurance. Because of its high glycemic index, it begins working immediately upon ingestion. The glycemic index calculates the rate at which a carbohydrate is absorbed. On a scale of one to 100, with 100 being the rate of absorption for a simple sugar such as glucose, the baked potato scores an impressive 98.

A garden-fresh vegetable salad paired with a baked potato makes a healthy, motivating meal. Be sure to eat the nutrient-rich skins, and instead of salt or butter, use salsa or guacamole to flavor the potato.

6. Reishi and Shiitake Mushrooms

Mushrooms, particularly Eastern varieties, revitalize the body. Various cultures consider them to contain the secrets of staying young. Reishi and shiitake mushrooms build resistance to stress by strengthening the immune system. They also provide key B vitamins to the liver and stimulate the adrenals with their high concentration of pantothenic acid. The common American button mushroom contains methionine, an amino acid high in sulphur. When combined with tofu, the result is a more complete protein.

7. Fruit Smoothies

Personally, I prefer fruit smoothies to energy bars. Compared to the dense, concentrated slabs, which are often a bit tough on the stomach and intestines, fruit juice is light, pure, and easily processed. When making smoothies, the most important ingredient is freshly squeezed seasonal fruits. I recommend watermelon in summer, orange and grapefruit in colder months. It's also essential to blend the fruit juice with protein-powered foods, such as brewer's yeast, bee pollen, soy protein, or spirulina. I like to add almond butter to my smoothies, and prescribe them to athletes in particular, as a pre- or post-event energy boost. My typical summertime fruit smoothie contains:

8 ounces of fresh squeezed watermelon juice
½ cup of papaya, cantaloupe, or watermelon
1 to 2 tbsp of almond butter
1 to 2 tbsp of brewer's yeast
1 tbsp Revita

For variety, substitute fresh squeezed orange juice, and use pineapple in place of the papaya or melon.

8. Seven-Grain Bread

The "staff of life," bread baked from whole grains, stabilizes blood sugar, detoxifies the liver, and invigorates the entire body. By providing an assortment of amino acids, complex carbs, enzymes, minerals, proteins, and vitamins, it nourishes the glands, digestive organs, musculoskeletal systems—you name it.

Seven-grain bread usually contains amaranth, millet, oat, quinoa, rice, rye, and wheat. Flourless, sprouted seven-grain bread is particularly rich in phytonutrients. Add organic almond butter to a seven-grain English muffin and wow! Energy without side effects. For extra flavor, spread a stamp-sized drop of pure honey on top.

Served with fresh fruit, seven-grain bread with almond butter makes an excellent breakfast. It also works well as a mid-meal pick-me-up. For lunch, I suggest avocado or hummus on either standard or flourless, sprouted seven-grain bread. Alternative sandwich spreads include the increasingly popular soy-based, egg-free "egg-salad" and dairy-free tofu cottage cheese. At dinner, enjoy seven-grain bread with a bowl of lentil or vegetable soup and a leafy green salad.

9. Veggie Burgers

Protein-rich vegetarian patties are made from an assortment of profoundly energizing plant foods. I suggest soy-based garden burgers, and recommend any sort of veggie burger over the powders used by athletes as protein supplements. Burgers give the stomach something to digest, but their nutrients are still quickly assimilated.

Falafel, millet, lentil, mushroom—a vegetarian burger exists for every taste, and many varieties are readily available in supermarkets and health food stores. Ideally, sandwich a veggie burger on seven-grain bread. Whole wheat or whole grain buns are also healthy options. A veggie burger makes for a substantial lunch or post-workout breakfast. For dinner, add a chlorophyll salad, seven-grain bread, and don't forget the Sunset Recharge's carrot juice. For an empowering alternative to spaghetti and meatballs, add chopped veggie burgers to a bowl of whole-grain pasta.

10. Tempeh

Tempeh is formed by fermenting tofu with *Rhizopus oligosporus*. In the process, tofu's inherent genistein and isoflavones are further enhanced, making tempeh a rich source of protein. Due to its chunky texture, tempeh is often mistaken for meat by many a novice sampling specialty dishes at Indonesian restaurants. Tempeh's high levels of phytonutrients help to detoxify the liver. Like all soy-based foods—tofu, miso, soy milk—tempeh fortifies the immune system. It protects the body from common and not-so-common viral infections and even helps to prevent cancer. For vegetarians, tempeh is one of the few sources of vitamin B_{12}. As such, it's a valuable addition to green vegetables, brown rice, and whole grain, udon, or rice noodles. Try tempeh burgers on seven-grain bread, or build a tasty vegetarian enchilada out of tempeh and mixed vegetables.

I guarantee that the high-performance plan outlined in Chapter 4 will increase your energy level. The top ten foods I've highlighted are all essential components of this diet, but many other vegetables—garlic, onions, parsley, and carrots, to name a few—also contain awesome healing powers. For a balanced nutritional program, it makes sense to rotate any and all beneficial phytonutrients. To complete this chapter, following are a few energizing items that just missed making the list:

11. Flaxseed

Flaxseed contains twenty-five anti-cancer compounds and is high in enzymes, fiber, and vitamin E. In a vegetarian diet, it is a key source of omega 3 fatty acids, and it has an overall anti-inflammatory effect. Add a couple of tablespoons of flaxseed, whole or crushed, to salads.

12. Sprouted Seeds

Fat-free sprouted seeds provide several phytonutrients and are bursting with enzymes. You can grow your own, without pesticides—it only takes a minute to water them each day. Varieties include: adzuki bean, baby greens, buckwheat lettuce, jumbo alfalfa, mung bean, and red clover.

13. Dulse and Nori

These two high-enzyme sea vegetables provide trace minerals scarce on mainland soil. Both can be added to salads and soups, or used to wrap rice and vegetable dishes.

Synthetic herbicides, pesticides, fertilizers, and additives destroy the phytonutrients naturally found in organic foods. Heavily processed products may last longer on the shelf, but at what price? Choose your own personal longevity over the longevity of packaged goods, and stick with fresh, organic, whole, energizing smart foods. You'll be rewarded with positive food swings and physical vigor.

CHAPTER 11

GOOD FOR YOU
AND GOOD FOR YOUR LOVE LIFE:
THE TEN SEXIEST FOODS

Can cuisine be an aphrodisiac? Since the dawn of civilization, lovers from every culture and age have pursued the elusive connection between passion and the palate. In an effort to increase their sex drive, they've experimented with all kinds of foods. Some fruits and vegetables were considered to be sexual because their shape resembled that of the reproductive organs: bananas, for example, or asparagus. Others, like the succulent peach, were lauded for their erotic texture. Still others—pumpkin seeds or almonds—earned a reputation for enhancing fertility.

Served in a sexually charged atmosphere—before a roaring fireplace, accompanied by the sultry strains of slow jazz—a flavorful, satisfying meal can entice all the senses. Even the upright Encyclopedia Britannica admits as much: "The visual satisfaction of appetizing food, the olfactory stimulation of their pleasing smells and the tactile gratification afforded the oral mechanisms by rich savory dishes can be conducive to sexual expression." Put in plain English, food can be a big turn-on.

When we are attracted to someone, all of our senses come alive: sight, smell, sound, taste, and touch. Exciting meals also arouse these feelings. Eating can be a sensual experience in and of itself, and specific foods can act as nutritional aphrodisiacs, heightening desire and the capacity for sexual pleasure.

By the same token, certain foods can also dampen sexual appetite. Contrary to popular conceptions, juicy red meat, soft raw oysters, heavy red wine, and rich chocolate desserts are **anaphrodisiacs** likely to leave you lethargic after a large meal. High-fat, high-protein foods may send you straight to bed . . . but only because your body feels so tired.

You snooze, you lose.

For example, milk, cheese, and turkey meat all contain proportionately high amounts of the sleep-inducing amino acid tryptophane. That's good news for insomniacs, but for those of us interested in revving up the libido, it's time to rethink our philosophy of sexy foods.

Before I discuss the leading nutritional aphrodisiacs, I want to clarify that the purpose of this chapter is to concentrate on the chemistry of love, as opposed to the chemistry of sex. As adults, we all know there is love without sex, and sex without love, but I'm interested in creating an integrated experience, one in which food helps to enhance positive sexual and spiritual emotions. I want to reach your heart and touch your soul. When sexuality, spirituality, intellect, and emotions are in balance, each area of your life benefits the other. The following information about sexual and sensual food swings is intended to strengthen the bond between two soulful, emotionally connected and committed lovers. It should not be regarded as a means of manipulation, deception, or control. In fact, such subversive attempts have a tendency to backfire: An unbalanced sex life, out of synch with spirituality and emotions, can, over time, depress the immune system and increase your susceptibility to disease.

I admit it. I believe in love. And I believe that lovemaking can dynamically enrich the relationship between two mutually respectful soul-mates. My Top Ten Sexiest Foods are my gift to those already in a meaningful emotional and spiritual partnership, and as enticing as all the foods are, none can take the place of the hottest ingredient of all, real love.

There are also a lot of single folks out there—those who, for one reason or another, choose celibacy, or have yet to meet the soul with whom they truly click. I haven't forgotten about you! Don't buy into the misbegotten notion that eating anaphrodisiacs will soothe your frustrated sexuality—these foods, such as the red meat and chocolate sweets I mentioned above, will undermine your general health. So even if you think they can't be applied to your life at present, read on to learn of the many fringe benefits of truly sexy foods.

THE SCIENCE OF SEXUAL NUTRITION

The emerging field of sexual nutrition studies how food affects the body's sexual response—both emotionally and physically. Dietary deficiencies and imbalances, combined with exhaustion and stress, are often diagnosed as causes of low sex drive. Burnout disables the pituitary-thyroid-adrenal axis, upsetting normal neuro-endocrine activity and eliminating sexual desire.

In general, the lighter the food, the more alkaline the meal, the better the body's sexual functioning. Heavy meals overload the lymph system and digestive organs. This glut slows down the body and hinders sexual performance. On the contrary, a light, mucus-free diet promotes sexual vitality, endurance, and appeal.

Pheromones are the body's naturally emitted, barely detectable, hormonal fragrances that attract and arouse. Specific nutrients—I've termed them "nutrimones"—can have a similar effect, simultaneously calming the nerves and activating the sex glands. What are these wonder nutrients, capable of boosting the libido, increasing sexual stamina, and improving performance?

Vitamin E, magnesium, potassium, and zinc are all essential to regulating hormones. L-arginine and gamma hydroxy butyrate (GHB) also impact sexual chemistry. And vitamin B_3, also known as niacin, increases blood flow to the pelvic organs and promotes erection.

It's the combination of such nutrients and their enzymes that determines food's ability to enhance sexual functioning. Each food item has its own chemistry, and some contain higher amounts of nutrimones than others. Eating the right foods as part of a high-performance diet, exercising regularly, and effectively managing stress all will contribute to your sexual vitality. Mind-body balance rejuvenates the sex glands.

ASPARAGUS SPEARS AND ARTICHOKE HEARTS

I mentioned earlier that, for centuries, food has been associated with sexuality. To this day, much of the folklore persists, or has been adapted to fit our culture. The medieval "Doctrine of Signatures" claimed that plants could be used to heal the body parts they resembled (which explains how asparagus spears and artichoke hearts got their sexy reputation!). Although the spuriousness of the edict may seem obvious in our supposedly advanced age, to its credit, it does get the imagination going. As you review the list of The Ten Sexiest Foods, think about the relationship between food and your love life.

THE TEN SEXIEST FOODS

1. CELERY
2. ASPARAGUS AND ARTICHOKE
3. AVOCADO
4. ONIONS AND TOMATOES (SALSA)
5. ALMONDS
6. PUMPKIN AND SUNFLOWER SEEDS
7. ROMAINE LETTUCE
8. WHOLE GRAIN BREADS
9. FRUITS AND NUTS
10. CHILIES, HERBS, AND SPICES

1. Celery

Awed by his powers, the ancient Romans dedicated celery to the god Pluto. Their folklore had it that " . . . if women knew what celery did to men, they would go and get some from Paris to Rome." In the Middle Ages, couples looked to celery when they wanted to give birth to a boy, with the pregnant wife placing a stalk underneath her pillow each night.

For men interested in attracting women, celery is the ultimate nutritional pheromone. It's as close as you can get to a spray-on aphrodisiac. High in androsterone, a potent male hormone, it also includes an excellent combination of essential minerals, enzymes, trace elements, and vitamins A, B, and C.

Add celery to salads and use it to garnish any vegetable entrée. Get your juices flowing with a carrot-celery shake or snack on celery stalks spread with unsalted almond butter. Of course, celery sticks make the perfect edible utensil when tasting dips.

2. Asparagus and Artichoke

In the 19th century, brides were served asparagus as part of their prenuptial dinner, to prepare them for their wedding night. Long considered an erotic symbol for its firm, bulbous stalks, asparagus combines invigorating chlorophyll with assorted minerals and enzymes. It's best when steamed, then tossed in a salad or paired with a baked potato.

Because of their shape and soft, petal-like, layers, artichokes have been associated with female genitalia. They contain many of the same nutrimones as asparagus, and the heart can be steamed, lightly grilled in olive oil, or peeled and added to salads.

3. Avocado

The avocado has a royal heritage: The pre-Colombian culture of the Maya believed that a tenth-century princess in what is now Mexico tasted the first fruit of its kind. The Aztecs used avocados, or *aguacate* (which actually derives from the Nahuatl word for testicle), as a sexual stimulant, and rubbed it into their hair for strength and luster.

Eating an avocado can be an extremely sensual experience. Its smooth, creamy texture is wonderful on the tongue. Once swallowed, its unsaturated fatty acids lubricate the glands, and its high percentage of vitamin E balances hormones. Try sliced avocado on seven-grain bread, or mash it into a flavorful guacamole and enjoy it with celery sticks or organic chips.

4. Onions and Tomatoes

Both onions and tomatoes have earned a reputation as aphrodisiacs, so watch out for that salsa! But it's not just native South Americans who are aware of the power of the pungent root vegetable and juicy vine fruit. In France, newlyweds were served onion soup the morning after their nuptials to replenish their libidos after a night of lovemaking. Both Hindu texts and Greek folklore refer to onions as sexual stimulants. In the days of the pharaohs, Egyptian priests were forbidden to eat onions because of their potential to arouse the sensual spirits within.

Called the "apple of love" by the French, the tomato, with its plump, flushed skin, brings to mind all sorts of sexual imagery. The phytonutrients in tomatoes have a phenomenal impact on sexual fluids, and the lycopene content may be responsible for the fruit's favorable influence on the prostate gland.

Spice up your diet with fresh salsa and organic chips. Use salsa on baked potatoes, in place of butter and salt. Serve pasta with a fresh tomato-basil sauce, and toast whole grain dough with tomatoes, onions, and mushrooms for an invigorating vegetarian pizza.

5. Almonds

The almond contains a magnificent blend of vitamins, minerals, enzymes, amino acids, and natural oils. Rich in calcium, magnesium, vitamin E, and zinc, its high alkaline content keeps sex glands healthy by preventing acid corrosion and protecting the organs. (When the prostate, seminal vesicle, or ovaries undergo acidic degeneration, sexual performance can be adversely affected.)

Warm almond-sesame milk acts as a relaxing aphrodisiac. It's also an excellent source of calcium for pregnant or breast-feeding women. To prepare:

Soak 1 cup of almonds in 2 cups of water overnight.
In the morning, retain the water, and blend the almonds with ½ cup of sesame seeds and 2 additional cups of water for 2 to 3 minutes on high speed.
Strain (the pulp can be used when baking bread) and return nut milk to blender.
Add 1 teaspoon of vanilla.
Add 1 tablespoon of honey or carob powder for flavor, of molasses for iron.
Add 1½ tablespoons of brewer's yeast for fiber.
Garnish with a sprinkle of cinnamon.

For fewer calories, substitute a banana for the honey and blend along with the nuts.

Almond butter, smooth or crunchy, makes a tasty pre-sex appetizer when spread on celery sticks. It also adds taste to whole grain toast, sesame crackers, and brown rice cakes. The morning after, chopped almonds can be added to whole grain cereal in order to replenish spent nutrients. To amplify the crunch, keep almonds refrigerated in an airtight container.

6. Pumpkin and Sunflower Seeds

The amino acids in pumpkin and sunflower seeds add crunch and protein punch to leafy green salads, fruit salads, and cereals. On their own, they make a handy snack. Because of their high concentration of zinc and unsaturated fatty acids, the seeds have traditionally been used to treat prostate dysfunction. Pumpkin pie, normally associated with such wholesome family holidays as Thanksgiving, also has a devilish side as an aphrodisiacal dessert.

7. Romaine Lettuce

Romaine rules the domain of the vegetable world. It is king of the lettuces. Caesar believed so strongly in its therapeutic powers that he erected a statue in its honor—hence his namesake salad.

Romaine lettuce contains an incredible balance of enzymes, minerals, vitamins, and, of course, chlorophyll. The darker the leaf, the greater its nutrimone content. Romaine should be a staple ingredient of any green salad. Add protein with pumpkin and sunflower seeds. A sexy dinner might consist of carrot-celery juice, followed by a Caesar salad and a main course of capellini pasta with fresh tomato-basil sauce. Top vegetarian enchiladas with salsa and serve alongside a Caesar salad, or use romaine in a classic Greek salad of tomatoes, red onions, and olives.

8. Whole Grain Breads

Seven-grain bread is very sexy, and toasting further enhances the crunch and flavor of its various elements, bringing the sensuality of this "staff of life" to its peak. Combined with other high-performance foods, whole grain bread is guaranteed to give you a below-the-belt charge. Add peanut butter, rich in niacin, and a sandwich really hits the spot. Spreads of avocado, almond butter, chickpeas, or garbanzo beans also put the libido back in business. (In ancient times, stallions were fed garbanzo beans to up their stud potential.) For a Middle Eastern pocket-style bite, add hommus to whole grain pita and season with tabbouleh (made from nutrimone-rich tomatoes and chopped green parsley). Or couch falafel burgers in whole-grain buns. Sometimes you only have five minutes to prepare lunch, and these whole grain sandwiches nurture, nourish, and stimulate.

9. Fruits and Nuts

Since time eternal, in the most poetic and profane terms, fruits and nuts have symbolized sexuality. The arc of a fruit—resulting from pollination, being plucked at its peak, then devoured in all of its sweet, sticky decadence—is undeniably erotic. Although modern mythology blames an apple on the tree of knowledge, historians wonder if it wasn't really quince, a hard, yellow fruit cultivated in the Mediterranean, that Eve used to lure Adam. In about 300 B.C., Theophrastos referred to quince as the "golden apple" of Hesperides (the nymphs), and because of its texture, scent, and color, the ancient Greeks attributed the fruit to Aphrodite, goddess of love. In some cultures, tradition states that eating quince at a wedding feast will help to ensure a satisfying love life.

Because of their shape and blushing coloration, berries have always been regarded as highly erotic. The Ancient Greeks enjoyed clusters of grapes at their hedonistic orgies. In Shakespeare's tragedy, Othello gives Desdemona a handkerchief embroidered with strawberries. Strawberry wine is reputed to be a love potion, while cherries represent a very specific part of the female anatomy. And no discussion of nutritional aphrodisiacs would be complete without mentioning the Coco-de-Mer. Commonly called the "double coconut," it is the largest fruit in the plant world and can weigh up to 50 pounds. Notorious for its shocking resemblance to the vulva and clitoris, Coco-de-Mer is a sought-after aphrodisiac. The jellylike interior of the fruit only affirms its reputation.

Nuts share an equally erotic history. In ancient Rome, walnuts were used in fertility rites, and they've maintained their popularity as an aphrodisiac in Italy and France. But pine nuts may rival walnuts as sexual stimulants. From the Mediterranean to the Far East, pine nuts have been celebrated for their potency. At around 100 B.C., the Roman sage Reatimus recommended pine nuts with pepper, mustard, and onions as a means of increasing sexual performance. Galen, a physician in ancient Greece, advised that pine nuts be paired with honey to enhance desire. The "Perfumed Garden" of Arabian folklore frequently refers to pine nuts as sexual tonics.

When it comes to incorporating fruits and nuts into your high-performance diet, you really can't go wrong. Add nuts to salads, pasta, and brown rice. Eat fruit at breakfast, as a snack, and as dessert. The exacting combinations of amino acids, enzymes, minerals, and vitamins make fruits and nuts complete proteins and even more complete aphrodisiacs. Whether it be peaches, cherries, or grapes, walnuts, almonds, or pine nuts, they revitalize your sexual chemistry and give you a warm glow.

10. Chilies, Herbs, and Spices

Spicy cayenne and a high content of vitamin C stimulate circulation, making chili a piquant aphrodisiac. Add beans—black or pinto—for protein. Other sexy spices and herbs include:

- **Mustard** increases the secretory potential of your sex glands and, like chili, has a stimulating effect on circulation.
- **Damiana** is the classic female sex tonic. It invigorates a woman's reproductive drive.
- **Fennel**, taken in small amounts, benefits sex drive in both genders.
- **Ginseng** is the male counterpart to damiana, but it can be used by women, too. Chinese Panax and Siberian are the best types for men.
- **Royal jelly** rejuvenates the body as a whole.
- **Saffron** has a reputation for charging up the sex hormones. It's also conducive to laughter.
- **Vanilla beans** work against sexual inertia and nurture the nervous system.

In this and the previous chapter, I've taken a proactive stance, listing my top energizing and sex-enhancing foods. With these nutritional tools in mind, let's go on the defense, and identify the SAD (Standard American Diet) items that deplete energy, decrease metabolic function, and exhaust the body.

CHAPTER 12

THE FATIGUE FACTOR:
AVOIDING THE TEN MOST TIRING FOODS

These days, everybody seems to be tired all the time. Our schedules are packed, we don't get enough sleep, and stress affects all areas of our existence. Certain exhausting factors are beyond our control, and at different points in life, we have to work extra hard just to keep it together. Maybe you're a new parent with a fitful baby. Maybe after you clock off work, you go straight to night school, where you're earning an advanced degree. Maybe you've just started your own business, and you spend every waking hour at the office. Whatever your circumstance, the important thing is to help yourself. Healthy foods that can keep us energized are at our disposal, yet so often we turn to the junk that gives us a short-term kick but ultimately burns us out.

Avoid foods that cause fatigue.

Fatigue can have many faces—physical, emotional, spiritual, professional—but the good news is, by positively altering body chemistry, high-performance nutrition can help them all. Contrarily, fast food causes dietary fatigue which, over time, damages organs and debilitates metabolism. To complicate matters, emotional food swings, such as compulsive overeating and bingeing, also contribute to fatigue. Exhaustion, stress, poor nutrition—it's all knotted up together. A steady diet of smart food, however, can untangle the mess.

THE ALMIGHTY LIVER

Eating the wrong foods results in liver stress. Harmful toxins and deleterious anti-nutrients hit the organ hard. High-fat, high-protein, rich, sweet, or acidic foods—and, of course, alcohol—are the most common culprits. They overload and agitate the liver, thereby interfering with its normal functioning. Thus provoked, the poor liver responds by secreting excess amounts of bile.

Ordinarily, bile lubricates and purifies the digestive, lymphatic, and circulatory systems to keep them running smoothly. By flushing out toxins, it prevents the organs from premature oxidation. In fact, I consider the liver to be the body's central biochemical organ. It is constantly processing, inactivating, and detoxifying dietary input. But when the liver is overwhelmed with anti-nutrients and acidic toxins, it reacts to the stress by producing additional bile. As the organ struggles against the assault and tries to bring the toxic load under control, chemicals back up in the bloodstream and tissues.

Think of it as a plumbing problem: Between the flood of excess bile in the digestive system and the clog of chemicals in the bloodstream, the body becomes sluggish and cranky. That's why crabby, ill-tempered types are described as "bilious."

DON'T POLLUTE

Liver stress results *from* dietary pollution, and results *in* foul bile and a fatty organ. When your liver is under toxic attack, you will not feel well. We've already established the connection between mind and body. The liver, of course, is an important part of that overall system. Liver dysfunction leads to adrenal dysfunction, pancreatic dysfunction, spleen dysfunction. It's a domino effect. Eventually, it causes damage to the pituitary-thyroid-adrenal axis, which then sends the body down the staircase of the three degrees of metabolic burnout I described in Chapter 3. Liver stress also negatively impacts the nervous system.

Your energy level is determined by the health of your metabolism, nerves, and hormones. Imagine, then, the harm done by emotionally induced oxidative food swings. They slow down metabolism with their overload of toxins and they produce reactions in the liver that ultimately imbalance the glandular and nervous systems. No wonder they cause fatigue—emotional, mental, and physical. By unbalancing body, including brain, chemistry, liver stress can also lead to depression. And depression itself is commonly characterized by inexplicable exhaustion. As always, it's a vicious swing cycle.

FOOD INTOLERANCE CAUSES FATIGUE

In addition to liver stress, food intolerances and allergies are another common cause of fatigue. The body is a tough machine, but at the cellular level, it's also very sensitive. As I explained in Chapter 4, anything from protein and starch to additives and colorings can cause an adverse reaction in the digestive system. Allergies vary according to the individual, but literally no body does well with toxic, commercial, poor-quality foods.

Of course, food intolerance also compounds liver stress: The liver is the organ forced to process the objective items.

Understand the cycle: The Standard American Diet causes dysfunctional food swings; dysfunctional food swings place stress on the liver. The more vulnerable the liver, the more fatigued the body and depressed the psyche. In turn, exhaustion and depression increase susceptibility to dysfunctional food swings. This graph illustrates the cycle of fatigue.

MENTAL FATIGUE OR MIND POWER?

The choice is yours: Mental and physical fatigue caused by liver stress undermine willpower and attitude. They interfere with self-confidence and kill your focus. It's tougher to resist temptation when you're tired—especially when you start fantasizing about how food could change your mood.

Mind power is the opposite of mental burnout. It is the first step toward realizing your thoughts. Mind power gives you the focus to:

1. Establish a positive attitude
2. Develop a positive belief system
3. Focus your expectations in a beneficial direction
4. Manifest your dreams

Mind power gives you dynamic will—the active intent to accomplish your dreams. High-performance nutrition feeds mind power. Dysfunctional, malnutritive, oxidative food swings debilitate it.

MIND POWER	MENTAL FATIGUE
Enthusiasm	Indifference
Pro-active	Reactive
Self-determination	Hesitancy
Strong-willed	Weak-willed
Self-confidence	Self-doubt
High self-worth	Low self-esteem
Self-discipline	Lack of discipline
Positive mental attitude	Negative mental attitude
Hustle	Laziness
Constructive belief systems	Destructive belief systems
Mental stamina	Mental quit
Interested in others	Self-absorbed
Optimistic	Depressed
Conviction	Purposelessness
Loving	Surviving
Letting go	Holding on

With practice, mind power can be learned. Meditation, affirmation, or prayer are all methods of promoting mind power. Train yourself by making a conscious effort to follow these seven steps:

1. Keep spirits high
2. Stay calm—easy does it
3. Take charge of your thought process
4. Regularly adjust attitude and lifestyle

5. Build self-confidence
6. Develop willpower
7. Commit to high-performance nutrition

The wrong foods drain mental energy. Without the support of the right fuel, mind power is restricted. And, as I have discussed extensively in previous chapters, mental fatigue sets up a cycle of dysfunctional food swings which, in turn, damage every other area of life—romantic and family relationships, finances, career, etc. To fortify nutritious food swings and resolve fear-based destructive belief systems, refer back to the **R.R.I.E.A. technique chart** I provide in Chapter 8 (see page 120).

Regardless of the issue, whether it's specifically about eating or it concerns larger lifestyle problems, the R.R.I.E.A. technique will put you in the driver's seat on the path to your own well-being. For example, if you feel trapped in a dead-end job or relationship, it takes good nutrition and a resilient mind to shift out of the comfort zone and confront the fears of failure, loneliness, rejection, and so on, that accompany major changes.

THE WAKE-UP CALL OF TIREDNESS

If you're truly tired, the last thing you want is a wake-up call, but it's the first thing you need. To a doctor of preventive medicine, fatigue is the most important warning sign. It opens the door for accurate assessment and rapid resolution of psychosomatic conflicts. Many of us dismiss fatigue—we say it's because we're getting older, or we're under stress, or our parents didn't have high energy levels, either. These are all excuses we use to avoid taking responsibility—step 1 of the R.R.I.E.A. technique—for our health management. To cling to the comfort zone, we have to keep up the denial.

I suggest that it's time to look at fatigue not as a burden to bear but a call to heed. Fatigue informs us that something's not working, and it invites us to find a new approach. It opens the door to healing our entire being—after all, emotional, mental, and physical exhaustion are all inextricably intertwined.

To combat fatigue through high-performance nutrition, not only is it essential to eat the energizing foods I described in Chapter 10. It's equally important to avoid the items that will tucker you out:

THE TEN MOST TIRING FOODS

1. EGGS
2. DAIRY PRODUCTS
3. CHOCOLATE AND SWEETS
4. WHITE BREAD AND BUTTER
5. BEEF AND PORK PRODUCTS
6. LOBSTER AND OTHER SHELLFISH
7. CANNED FRUIT
8. FRIED CHICKEN
9. SALTED CHIPS, NUTS, OR CRACKERS
10. ALCOHOL

1. Eggs

Even more so than milk products, eggs are mucus-forming, clogging the head, neck, and throat. Eggs cause stagnation in the lymph system and lead to back-ups in the liver, spleen, and biliary plumbing. Albumin, the protein found in eggs, is a common allergen, and particularly affects children, who often suffer from recurrent ear infections.

Rule out foods that include egg whites, egg yolks, or albumin, and read labels carefully to find these hidden sources of egg products:

Globulin
egg lysozyme
ovomucoid
ovovitellin
livetin
ovoglobulin
ovotransferrin
vitellin

Try tofu instead of eggs—it offers the equivalent in protein, without the mucus.

2. Dairy Products

Milk and dairy products are high-fat foods that make the mind and body sluggish. As with eggs, dairy products can induce drowsiness within ten minutes of consumption, and their lethargic effects can last for up to five hours. Milk protein is another common food allergen, and lactose intolerance is a widespread dietary disorder. Eliminating dairy is a necessary step for anyone afflicted with recurrent bronchitis, tonsillitis, sinusitis, colitis, candida, bladder infections, or any form of indigestion. Moreover, dairy further compromises a suppressed immune system, and so should not be eaten by anyone treating rheumatoid arthritis, asthma, HIV, lupus, or multiple sclerosis.

Common forms of dairy include all variations of milk, cheese and spreads, ice cream, mayonnaise, and yogurt. On product labels, look for these hidden sources of dairy:

acidophilus milk
casein
curds
galactose
ghee
lactate
lactoalbumin
lactoglobulin
lactose
malted milk
potassium caseinate
whey

Low-fat and rennetless dairy products are safer alternatives which still offer the same creamy sensation we so often crave. Almond, rice, and soy milks and cheeses, for example, provide the emotional pleasure of traditional dairy without the accompanying fatigue.

3. Chocolate and Sweets

Chocolates and sweets take the cake, so to speak, as the most popular comfort foods. But, as explained in Chapter 3, refined white sugars wreak havoc on the pancreas, liver, adrenals, and blood system. Chocolates, candies, cookies, and the like all contribute to the highs and lows of fluctuating blood sugar levels—the sugar cycle, remember? Few dysfunctional food swings are as exhausting. Substitute fruit with nuts or whole-grain toast spread with almond butter and you'll satisfy your sweet tooth without suffering the consequences of fatigue.

4. White Bread And Butter

It just doesn't seem like dinner without that basket of rolls and the little tub or butter on the side, does it? (Not to mention the pre-meal sodas and cocktails, all of which decrease energy.) But butter (which technically belongs above with its fellow dairy products, but on a more instinctive level can never be separated from its counterpart, bread) is mucus-forming, and refined white carbohydrates cause functional hypoglycemia. Commonplace low blood sugar is characterized by the come-and-go fatigue that directly corresponds to the timing of meals.

White flour can cause serious liver stress. In fact, any refined carbohydrates, from white rice to macaroni to breakfast cereals to flour tortillas, will produce the same soporific effect as white bread. Try whole grains instead, and use olive oil in place of butter.

5. Beef and Pork Products

We're bombarded by so many ads for burgers and steaks that just watching TV makes me weary. Animal proteins are high in saturated fats, which clog the circulatory and digestive systems and cause liver and pancreatic stress. Furthermore, animal proteins are acid- and mucus-forming, resulting in additional stress to the liver, spleen, and kidneys. The amount of nitrites, nitrates, and artificial chemicals in many of these mass-produced foods are enough to terrify your liver. Any of these effects in and of itself is tiring: Imagine how exhausting it must be when they're all combined in one dish! Think back to the last time you indulged in a bacon cheeseburger. How long did it take before you began to feel tired?

Avoid meat before any significant social, athletic, or even sexual event. If you don't, your body will be too busy digesting to have any energy left for anything else.

6. Lobster and Other Shellfish

In my part of the country, southern California, and also down in nearby Mexico, seafood, especially lobster, crab, shrimp, and other shellfish, is a very popular part of the regional cuisine. However, not unlike animal proteins, lobster and shellfish are high in fatigue-inducing saturated fats. The cholesterol content in shellfish is also substantial. Since these creatures are scavengers, they tend to ingest other pollutants at the bottom of the ocean: heavy metal contamination, of mercury in particular, damages the liver. It's worth a note here that it's always safer to eat lower on the food chain: By the time you get to the top, too many toxins may have infiltrated.

7. Canned Fruit

The sky-high sucrose content of the artificially sweetened juices and chemical preservatives that bathe canned fruits make them no different than refined white carbs. Many salad bars, cafeterias, and diners mix canned fruits with sliced cantaloupe or pineapple in their supposed diet dishes and healthy desserts. When you eat out, be certain that the fruit platter you order is fresh. If possible, wait until you get home and make your own bowl of fruit and nuts.

8. Fried Chicken

Chicken's high saturated fat and acidic content, compounded by frying, make this meat toxic to the liver. Chicken is also stressful to the pancreas and it upsets hormonal balance, increasing the risk of everything from arthritis to breast or prostate cancer. The Conspiracy promotes chicken as a healthy meat. Don't believe the TV commercial hype.

9. Salted Chips, Nuts, and Crackers

Salty foods temporarily satisfy a craving for stimulation, they encourage the hand-to-mouth reflex, and they're tough to avoid—imagine a party without potato chips. The next time you eat a bunch of salted nuts, popcorn, or crackers, mark how quickly your mood and energy level shift. And watch out for those white chips.

Salted snacks upset the body's delicate balance between potassium and sodium, and they stress the kidneys, liver, and nervous system. But with a proper potassium-to-sodium ratio, maintained in part by unsalted chips and roasted or raw almonds and cashews, body tissues thrive.

10. Alcohol

Alcohol is the most overrated drug on the market. Because it's legal, we forget that it's lethal. Alcohol attacks the liver and causes reactive hypoglycemia. Although social drinkers consider champagne, wine, and scotch as mood lifters, alcohol is actually a depressant that inhibits the central nervous system. Need proof? Quit drinking for an entire month—or at least 21 days. Then, when you have your first glass of wine, or bottle of beer, or sugar-spiked cocktail, time how long it takes for you to start feeling tired. If you limit your alcohol intake to just a drink or two at special celebrations, you'll be able to maintain your energy level.

Eating right is a proactive part of improving your health. *Not* eating *wrong* is equally important. (In the next chapter, I'll discuss how to overcome the anxiety and depression that often result from dysfunctional-food-swing-induced fatigue.) Teach yourself to avoid the foods that drain you. It will simplify and stabilize your life.

CHAPTER 13

FIGHTING BACK WITH SMART FOOD:
THE TEN BEST ANTI-DEPRESSING, MOOD-LIFTING, ANXIETY-FIGHTING FOODS

When is the last time you stopped to wonder how we all got so mixed up in this high-stress lifestyle? Indeed, modern telecommunications have made the world a more efficient place. And in response, our own rate of performance has increased. Not just our machines, but we, too, are expected to react better, stronger, faster. The biotechnology of human behavior has taken quantum leaps in just the past two decades, and already such advances as the fax machine are becoming obsolete.

Today, time-saving and multi-tasking are our top priorities, tailored toward materialistic ends: More work, more money, more stuff. Rush, rush, rush. Like robots, we adhere to our self-imposed routines: home to work, back and forth, with lots of errands in between: bill-paying and parent-teacher conferences, Friday nights at the bar and Saturday mornings at the kids' soccer games.

Some culture critics have compared the stress of our plugged-in lifestyle to that of living in the wilderness. It's survival of the fittest, with machines as weapons. But there's a price tag on all this high-tech hyper-productivity.

The more we focus on our financial and professional performance, the more likely it is that our emotional needs get neglected. As a consumeristic society, we have more than ever, so why are we lonely, anxious, and depressed?

Anxiety and depression are symptoms of an ailing emotional life, and are often brought on by the pressure to keep up 'the modern-day pace. Excess stress, internalized frustrations, endless distractions, and unmet emotional needs lead to anxiety. Anxiety immediately attacks the nervous system and strains the cardiac muscles. Over time, it leads to depression, which drains energy levels and muddies mental focus. This spiritual and emotional deficit is affecting larger numbers of young people, too—contributing to everything from attention disorders in kids to premature menopause or impotence in adults. Today, nearly thirty million Americans take antidepressant medication.

FIGHT BACK WITH SMART FOOD

If food can energize (Chapter 10), and food can improve your sex life (Chapter 11), doesn't it stand to reason that food can also counter depression? If the wrong foods can cause stress (Chapter 4), doesn't it stand to reason that the right foods can fight it?

Anxiety and depression need to be handled. They are ever-present conditions of contemporary life. They can't be cured, but they can be controlled. We Americans often approach our more tangible breakdowns—whether it's a broken ankle or bad case of acne—with aggressive treatments. We've been taught to treat physical, visible problems with all sorts of remedies. But we drastically underestimate the importance of emotional well-being. We think that if we just ignore it, it will eventually go away. When it doesn't, we turn to doctors for quick-fix drug prescriptions. But, as I discussed in Chapter 7, I am a big believer in the maxim "an ounce of prevention is worth a pound of cure."

Like fatigue, anxiety and depression can be considered wake-up calls, warning signs. Your mind, body, and spirit are trying to tell you something is wrong. They signal the need for change. As you acknowledge anxiety and depression, take into account the following four factors:

1. *The choice is yours.* You can heal emotional disorders, or you can medicate them. In my professional, medical opinion, taking prescription drugs is

the path of least resistance. Anti-anxiety agents can further numb upsetting feelings, turning you into an **emotional zombie**. Directly addressing and healing the dysfunctions requires strength and courage. It's a longer process, but it's one that will reward you with a profound understanding of self.

2. *Nutrition impacts body chemistry.* Emoto-Nutrition (Chapter 9) is a very real, very practical part of nutritional healing. Nutrient deficiencies and bio-chemical imbalances can instigate or aggravate anxiety and depression.

3. *The right food choices create therapeutic food swings that calm anxiety and lift depression.*

4. *The wrong food choices create dysfunctional food swings that exacerbate anxiety and deepen depression.* At this point, you're quite familiar with the culprits: They're many of the same foods behind fatigue:

- ice cream and other fatty dairy products
- candy, cookies, and other sugary sweets
- soda and other sugary soft drinks
- packaged cereals
- bacon, hamburgers, and other beef and pork products
- caffeine
- alcohol
- white crackers and cheese
- salted chips, nuts, and pretzels

THREE DEGREES OF DEPRESSION AND ANXIETY

Remember the three degrees of burnout I discussed in Chapter 3? Anxiety and depression, too, are degenerative. There are **mild, moderate,** and **advanced** levels of these **emotional disorders**. Milder forms tend to be situational and short-lived. They may begin when, instead of taking **responsibility** for a specific problem, **experiencing** the unpleasant emotions, and taking **action** to counter them, an individual instead treats him- or herself with SAD (Standard American Diet) stuff, and swallows feelings down with the junk. Such episodic or cyclical bouts can almost always be healed with natural herbs and healthy foods. **First-degree depression** does not usually require the supervision of a qualified counselor or psychologist. It certainly **does not merit medication**.

Moderate, or **intermediate**, forms of anxiety and depression are more troublesome. Even though they can also often be traced back to dysfunctional food swings, the depth and duration of the disorder are more extensive. Although you can still treat moderate anxiety and/or depression with nutritional remedies, at this second-degree stage, I believe a competent counselor, one who specializes in behavioral and personality dysfunctions, is needed to evaluate the problem. Therapy helps to sort out suppressed emotional and spiritual issues.

Advanced anxiety or depression demands the attention of a qualified psychiatrist in addition to talk therapy, nutritional healing, and vitamin supplementation. In my experience, patients suffering from extreme anxiety and/or depression are candidates for prescriptive agents. But individuals in the first or second stage of anxiety or depression can be healed with top-notch emotional counseling and high-performance foods. No drugs.

The purpose of this chapter is to identify the therapeutic foods that naturally alleviate anxiety and depression. Before I outline them, let's take a closer look at the metabolic patterns of these emotional disorders. It will help to explain how certain foods can positively alter biochemistry.

DEPRESSION: THE COMMON COLD OF MODERN PSYCHIATRY

These days, depression is as common as a cold. Typical symptoms include a loss of interest in activities, an inability to experience pleasure, poor job performance, memory loss, and a low level of energy. Sufferers feel hopeless. They withdraw from social situations, their outlook is pessimistic, and they are easily irritated.

Nutritional deficiencies, undiagnosed food allergies, alcohol abuse, functional hypoglycemia, liver disease, candida, PMS, neurological imbalances, suppressed immune systems, prescription drugs, and environmental toxicity: A variety of metabolic factors contribute to depression. For example, alcohol inhibits the central nervous system and aggravates functional hypoglycemia. Between alcohol-depressed nerves and the anxiety produced by the sugar cycle, it's a recipe for emotional disaster. Coffee is another culprit. Caffeine in and of itself irritates nerves and can cause headaches. Add milk, with its high-fat content and mucus-forming capacity, and sugar, which gives the body a false boost of energy, and a café au lait equals a common clinical triad behind depression. Think about how tough it is on the body: You have a couple of cocktails with dinner, followed by coffee and dessert. In the span of an hour, you've consumed an assortment of contradictory elements that send the body on a roller-coaster ride of peaks and crashes.

Above all, hormones influence mood. Stress-related thyroid or adrenal dysfunctions trigger depression—and because depression stifles the thyroid gland and depletes its hormones, many depressed people wind up overweight (a healthy thyroid is essential to an efficient metabolism). Overloaded adrenals result in decreased levels of norepinephrine and DHEA (dehydroepiandrosterone), the lack of which negatively impacts moods.

Furthermore, there's a direct relationship between the absence of three specific amino acids—**tryptophane, phenylalanine**, and **tyrosine**—and the appearance of depression. A deficiency of specific vitamins, such as B_6 and **folic acid**, can also contribute to the problem.

LOW SEROTONIN

Serotonin, an important neurotransmitter, is believed by many medical authorities to be responsible for stabilizing or elevating mood (higher amounts promote positive feelings, while lower amounts result in irritability and depression). Others consider it a natural tranquilizer. As part of the brain's ongoing chemistry, tryptophane converts to serotonin. Therefore, diets deficient in this amino acid result in bodies deficient in the soothing neurotransmitter. Commonly prescribed antidepressants tap into this particular metabolic pathway and increase levels of serotonin in the brain.

To avoid the use of prescription antidepressants and still treat the disorder, it's important to understand that diet affects serotonin levels. For example, reactive hypoglycemia and cigarette-smoking decrease serotonin production, while excess consumption of protein, alcohol, carbohydrates, and sugars interferes with the conversion of the amino acid to the neurotransmitter.

Because tryptophane is a precursor to serotonin, eating foods high in tryptophane offers a viable nutritional alternative to standard Prozac or Zoloft therapy. Doctors of preventive medicine prescribe 100–200 mg of 5-HTP (5-hydroxytryptophane, a compound produced in the conversion of tryptophane to serotonin) three times a day to treat depression. It acts as a nutritional supplement, it is better absorbed by the body than straight trypto-phane, and it not only elevates serotonin levels but also increases the amount of other endorphins and neurotransmitters that are often low in patients suffering from depression.

By choosing foods high in tryptophane, and supplementing your diet with 5-HTP, you can treat depression without prescription drugs. Side effects are practically non-existent—occasional nausea or digestive dysfunction.

THE TOP TEN FOODS HIGH IN TRYPTOPHANE

1. ALFALFA SPROUTS
2. BEETS
3. BROCCOLI
4. CARROTS
5. CAULIFLOWER
6. CELERY
7. ENDIVE
8. SPINACH
9. TOFU AND SOYBEAN PRODUCTS
10. WATERCRESS

PHENYLALANINE AND TYROSINE: THE OTHER ANTIDEPRESSANT AMINO ACIDS

Previously, I mentioned three amino acids. Tryptophane, the first, plays a crucial role in emotional control because it is converted into mood-enhanc-ing serotonin. The second, phenylalanine, also converts into a natural anti-depressant, phenylethylamine (or PEA). PEA is found in many healthy foods. Apparently, touching, hugging, and other expressions of physical inti-macy also build up the body's PEA. Conversely, levels of this biogenic amine decline when two lovers terminate their relationship. Chocolate has a high level of PEA: As much as it's a comfort food, it does also fulfill a biochemi-cal craving on the part of the heartbroken!

Phenylalanine is an essential component in the brain's production of nor-epinepherine, a hormonal mood booster that is often depleted due to adre-nal stress. And in addition to promoting positive moods, phenylalanine decreases the rate at which endorphins and enkephalins are broken down. Because these are the brain's natural opiates, their extension helps to alleviate pain and prolong good moods.

THE TOP TEN FOODS HIGH IN PHENYLALANINE

1. ALMONDS
2. AVOCADOS
3. BEANS
4. PARSLEY
5. PEANUT BUTTER
6. PINEAPPLE
7. MISO SOUP
8. SPINACH
9. TOFU AND SOYBEAN PRODUCTS
10. TOMATOES

Phenylalanine is also sold in the form of a nutritional supplement called DLPA, or DL-phenylalanine. It can be taken in doses of 500 mg, twice daily. Those suffering from depression have lower endorphin levels, and DLPA aids in elevating them. For this reason, it is prescribed as a natural painkiller as well as a nutriceutical antidepressant.

Tyrosine, the third amino acid, also crosses the blood-brain barrier to counter depression. Just as phenylalanine supports the adrenals, tyrosine stimulates the thyroid (it helps out the adrenals, too) and works to stabilize blood sugar. To do so, it requires vitamin B_3, vitamin C, and folic acid to facilitate its conversion into norepinepherine and dopamine—another key neurotransmitter. Whenever stress factors into depression, tyrosine is the go-to amino acid. It corrects body chemistry by regulating the all-important P.T.A. axis.

THE TOP TEN FOODS HIGH IN TYROSINE

1. ALMONDS AND ALMOND BUTTER
2. APPLES
3. ASPARAGUS
4. AVOCADOS
5. CARROTS
6. PEANUT BUTTER

7. ROMAINE LETTUCE
8. SPINACH
9. TOFU AND SOYBEAN PRODUCTS
10. WATERMELON

Cucumbers, parsley, and watercress also contain tyrosine.

FOLIC ACID DEFICIENCY AND DEPRESSION

Folic acid is an important B complex vitamin and plays an active role in balancing brain chemistry. It nourishes the bloodstream and supports the immune system. Along with vitamin B_{12} and S-adenosylmethionine (or SAM, a derivative of the amino acid methionine), folic acid regulates neurotransmitters. It raises SAM levels, which, in turn, raise levels of serotonin and dopamine.

Some studies state that as many as 33 percent of depressed patients lack the nutrient. This is especially true for the elderly: 85 percent of the geriatric depressed population consumes insufficient amounts of folic acid. But folic acid deficiency is an unacceptable cause of depression, because so many high-performance foods contain copious amounts of it. For example, all leafy green vegetables and legumes bolster folic acid levels.

THE TOP TEN FOODS HIGH IN FOLIC ACID

1. ASPARAGUS
2. BEANS (GARBONZO, KIDNEY, MUNG, AND NAVY)
3. BREWER'S YEAST
4. BROCCOLI
5. KALE AND BEET GREENS
6. LENTILS AND BLACK-EYED PEAS
7. SPINACH
8. TOFU AND SOYBEAN PRODUCTS
9. WHEAT GERM
10. WHOLE WHEAT CEREALS AND BREADS

Other excellent sources of folic acid include: almonds, avocados, green beans, mustard greens, peanuts, split peas, and walnuts.

VITAMIN B₆ DEFICIENCY AND DEPRESSION

In the conversion of tryptophane to serotonin, vitamin B_6 is an essential co-factor, and therefore a B_6 deficiency will adversely affect the serotonin metabolism. B_6 imbalances are common in depressed women suffering from PMS or menopause. The nutrient can also be inactivated by hormones present in birth control or estrogen replacement medication. Compensate for B_6 shortages by stocking up on the following smart foods:

THE TOP TEN FOODS HIGH IN VITAMIN B₆

1. AVOCADOS
2. BANANAS
3. BEANS (GARBONZO, LIMA, NAVY, AND PINTO)
4. BREWER'S YEAST
5. BROWN RICE
6. LENTILS
7. SPINACH
8. SUNFLOWER SEEDS
9. TOFU AND SOYBEAN PRODUCTS
10. WALNUTS

Black-eyed peas, potatoes, and whole wheat flour are also good sources of vitamin B_6.

OMEGA-3 FATTY ACIDS AND HERBAL THERAPY

One final note: Omega-3 fatty acids also aid in the prevention of emotional disorders, and a deficiency can contribute to severe depression. The brain is the top source of fatty acids in the body, and it requires the omega-3s for optimal functioning. Add one or two tablespoons of flaxseed oil to green leafy vegetable salads to get the full complement of daily omega-3 fatty acids.

To treat mild and moderate forms of depression, herbal therapy, combined with a diet of the foods I've listed above, can be effective. I advise that the following herbal remedies be taken in the following dosages, along with 100 mg of 5-HTP, three times daily:

- Saint John's wort (.3% hypericin): 300 mg three times daily for those under 55
- Ginkgo biloba (24% ginkgo flavoglycosides): 60 mg three times daily for those over 55

ANTI-ANXIETY NUTRITIONAL TRANQUILIZERS

Those suffering from depression often find it difficult to muster up the energy to do much of anything, and they generally feel emotionally exhausted. If depression is characterized by lethargy of the mind, body, and soul, anxiety is all about tension. Anxious individuals are tightly wound, apprehensive, even panic-stricken. It's an unpleasant state, and we've become accustomed to medicating it with Valium or Xanax. Most physicians prescribe the popular tranquilizers to help patients who have difficulty sleeping, or who cannot stop worrying. What I personally fail to understand is, what good does it accomplish in the long run to numb real concerns with pharmaceuticals? How can anyone ever resolve troublesome issues if they're simply silenced?

The most that psychoactive drugs can do is momentarily calm anxiety. Nutritional tranquilizers, however, provide biochemical support while still allowing the sufferer to get to the cause—to confront crises, **experience** feelings, take **action**, and resolve conflict permanently. Instead of automatically turning to drugs, anxiety-prone individuals should first look to smart foods to soothe their nerves. The proper food swings are free of negative side effects, do not numb emotions, and do not cloud the thinking process.

No hangovers. No toxic residue to the liver. And the body does not build up a tolerance to smart food—it's not necessary to eat more and more tofu just to maintain peace of mind.

The dietary secret to alleviating and eliminating anxiety can be found in the mineral and vitamin content of anti-xyolitic foods. Magnesium, along with zinc and vitamins B_1, B_2, B_3, and B_6, keeps the wolves at bay. In addition, review the effects that functional hypoglycemia and LIAS (Chapter 9) have on dysfunctional food swings, and adjust your diet accordingly to further prevent anxiety.

MELLOW MAG

Magnesium has a sedative influence on the neuro-muscular system. It stills anxious souls. Irritability, edginess, grouchiness, and moodiness are all indicative of a magnesium deficiency. Those afflicted with fibromyalgia and other stress-related disorders, those who experience chronic tension in the neck and back muscles, and those generally nervous and fidgety will all greatly benefit from an increased intake of magnesium-rich foods.

THE TOP TEN FOODS HIGH IN MAGNESIUM

1. ALMONDS
2. AVOCADOS
3. BROWN RICE
4. CARROTS
5. LENTILS
6. ORANGE, GRAPEFRUIT, AND PINEAPPLE (CITRUS FRUITS)
7. POTATOES
8. ROMAINE LETTUCE AND DARK LEAFY GREEN VEGETABLES
9. SESAME SEEDS
10. TOFU AND SOYBEAN PRODUCTS

Other foods high in magnesium include: apricots, barley, corn, lima beans, mushrooms, peanut butter, and tomatoes. A fresh green salad with guacamole is an excellent source of the mineral.

THINK ZINC

Zinc is another miracle nutrient capable of calming ragged nerves. Along with magnesium, it helps to maintain the nervous system. Without the two minerals, anxiety is inevitable.

Alarmingly, many factors in our comprised environment disrupt the delicate alkaline mineral balance. Artificial fertilizers, pesticides, phosphorous-heavy soft drinks, and copper from water pipes are just a few of the varied causes of magnesium and zinc deficiencies. Alcohol, undiagnosed food intolerances and allergies, and stress also drain the body of minerals.

Supplement the magnesium-rich foods listed above with the following high-zinc items for a stable, alkaline, mineral content in the blood and tissues.

THE TOP TEN FOODS HIGH IN ZINC

1. ALMONDS
2. BRAZIL NUTS
3. GREEN PEAS
4. LIMA BEANS
5. OATS
6. PEANUTS
7. PECANS
8. PUMPKIN SEEDS
9. SPLIT PEAS
10. WHOLE WHEAT GRAINS

Black beans, carrots, parsley, potatoes, and walnuts will also increase dietary intake of zinc.

VITAMIN B₁: THIAMINE TIME

Thiamine, the first of the B vitamins, acts as an important cofactor in the operation of the enzyme thiamine-pyrophospate (TPP), which helps regulate carbohydrate metabolism, energy production, and nerve cell function. Additionally, thiamine potentiates the effects of acetylcholine, the central neurotransmitter responsible for the prevention of memory loss.

Ordinarily, thiamine, or vitamin B_1, insures that pyruvic acid is oxidized and converted into usable energy. But when the vitamin is deficient, pyruvic acid first accumulates, then is converted into lactic acid, which, of course, turns into lactate. For lactose-intolerant individuals, this buildup results in LIAS—Lactate-Induced Anxiety Syndrome (as explained in Chapter 9). Because it's essential to the efficiency of nerve endings and neurotransmitters, vitamin B_1 deficiency also leads to irritability.

Thiamine is extremely vulnerable to alcohol and sulfites. These toxins can inactivate the vitamin and cause all the aforementioned, anxiety-related side effects. To avoid the unnecessary angst, keep liquor consumption to a minimum and eat foods high in thiamine.

THE TOP TEN FOODS HIGH IN THIAMINE (VITAMIN B₁)

1. BREWER'S YEAST
2. BROWN RICE
3. MILLET
4. OATMEAL
5. PINE NUTS
6. PINTO BEANS
7. SPLIT PEAS
8. SUNFLOWER SEEDS
9. TOFU AND SOYBEAN PRODUCTS
10. WHEAT GERM

In general, legumes, nuts, whole wheat, and whole grains are all good sources of thiamine. Brazil nuts, macadamias, peanuts, and pistachios round out the list.

VITAMIN B₃: NIACINAMIDE, THE NERVE PROTECTOR

There are two components of vitamin B_3: niacin and niacinamide. Niacin contains enzymes that aid carbohydrate metabolism at the cellular level. It is an indispensable part of NAD and NADP enzyme systems, which guarantee that carbs are efficiently converted into fuel. Niacinamide has a Valium-like impact on nerves. A diet deficient in vitamin B_3 can cause the malnutritive condition pellagra, in which brain function deteriorates and ultimately ends in dementia.

Nourish your nervous system with these sources of niacinamide: barley, brewer's yeast, brown and wild rice, buckwheat, peas, peanuts, red chili peppers, sesame and sunflower seeds, rice bran and wheat bran, whole wheat and seven-grain breads.

VITAMIN B₆: THE POWER OF PYRIDOXINE

Thinking and memory require instant, precise communication from one nerve ending to another. **Glutamic acid** is the vital neurotransmitter that activates and transmits information from the rest of the body to the brain. It empowers quick thinking. **Gamma-aminobutyric acid**, or GABA, is the neurotransmitter that slows down the work of the activating excitatory glutamic acid. It has a sedative effect on the nervous system. When glutamic acid and GABA work in tandem, nerves remain calm and thinking clear.

GABA, the inhibitory neurotransmitter, is made from glutamic acid, the stimulatory neurotransmitter. Vitamin B_6, or pyridoxine, acts as a catalyst in this conversion, metabolizing glutamic acid. When there is a relative deficiency of B_6, an excess of glutamic acid is unopposed by lower-than-normal levels of GABA. Overstimulation and irritability can result. Whereas with adequate supplies of B_6, sufficient supplies of GABA are manufactured, and the nerves are consequently sedated. This is how, by extension, vitamin B_6 prevents anxiety.

Magnesium, the tranquilizing mineral, also works in conjunction with pyridoxine to alleviate nervous tension.

THE TOP TEN FOODS HIGH IN PYRIDOXINE (VITAMIN B_6)

1. AVOCADOS
2. BANANAS
3. BREWER'S YEAST
4. BROWN RICE
5. GARBONZO BEANS
6. LENTILS
7. PINTO BEANS
8. SUNFLOWER SEEDS
9. TOFU AND SOYBEAN PRODUCTS
10. WALNUTS

There's also a plentiful supply of vitamin B_6 in whole grains, whole wheat, and cruciferous vegetables.

Deficiencies in vitamin B_6 have been linked to asthma, autoimmune disorders, carpal tunnel syndrome, depression, heart conditions, kidney stones, PMS, and seizure disorders. The increase in the appearance of these ailments parallels the increase in B_6 antagonists present in prescription drugs and processed foods. Alcohol, birth control pills, hydrazine dyes, anti-tuberculosis isoniazid, and anti-hypertensive hydralazine are among the more common B_6 antagonists.

You are what you eat. Minerals, B vitamins, and amino acids can do everything from boosting serotonin to soothing nerves. Take encouragement from the knowledge that food can do so much to effectively eliminate anxiety and depression. A high-performance diet, combined with emotional and spiritual awareness, results in a happy, balanced life, free of mood-numbing pharmaceuticals.

PART 3

FOOD
PERSONALITIES

AS A DOCTOR OF preventive medicine, I rely on the healing power of food to help my patients get and stay well. In the process of treating thousands upon thousands of individuals, I've personally witnessed the proof in the proverb "you are what you eat." Taking this thought to the next level, I've also discovered that each food item has a personality of its own—a unique combination of distinctive characteristics. To maximize your own potential, match your personality to the foods that will most enhance it.

There are hundreds of common food items available at the supermarket, and each one offers a different emotional value: Some foods (such as the "Ten Sexiest" I listed in Chapter 11) will promote passion and vibrancy. Others cause crankiness and fatigue. All of us can benefit by experimenting with our diets—explore how diet can make you emotional, spiritual, sexy, or intellectually sharp. The previous two sections of *Food Swings* explained how food influences mood. The following five chapters can serve as a compendium, an alphabetized reference guide to the benefits of various fruits, vegetables, grains, legumes, nuts, and seeds. And one final note: My suggestions for combining foods are based not only on taste, but also on the body's optimal assimilation and digestion of nutrients.

CHAPTER 14
FRUIT PERSONALITIES

Fruits feature incredible healing properties. They're high in phytonutrients, enzymes, vitamins, and minerals. Regular fruit consumption has
been proven to protect against cancer and cardiac disease as well as premature aging and other degenerative disorders. Excellent sources of antioxidants, fruits are a classic high-fiber, low-fat food group. The icing on the
cake, so to speak, is that fruits are also sweet and satisfying. A fruit-based
breakfast is a staple of the Sunrise Cleanse (see Chapter 6), as part of a balanced, high-performance nutritional program.

**In order to maximize the metabolic benefits of fruits, make your
selections based on what is in season**. For example, focus on orange
juice in winter and watermelon juice in summer. And if you suffer from candidiasis, diabetes, or functional hypoglycemia, consult with a physician to
determine how much and what kind of fruit you should incorporate into your
nutritional program.

I prefer to classify fruits according to their acid content, and I assign them
to one of three categories:

A. Acid Fruits

B. Sub-acid Fruits

C. Alkaline Fruits

ACID FRUITS

ORANGES

Notable Personality Factors: Oranges have long been the icon of the citrus fruits. They promote alertness and confidence, increase energy levels, and invigorate. They brighten spirits, boost mental attitude, and bring hope. Fresh squeezed o.j. is an eye-opener. Oranges are also good for circulation—hence the daily glass of orange juice in the Sunrise Cleanse (See page 83).

Therapeutic and Healing Powers: The flavonoids and bioflavonoids in oranges, combined with their high vitamin C content, make the fruit a strong ally of the immune system. Individuals with a substantial intake of oranges have a much lower incidence of cancer. Oranges' assortment of phytonutrients and enzymes are of particular benefit to the prevention of upper respiratory infections. The fruit has a detergent action, loosening mucus in the upper respiratory passages (the exact opposite effect of mucus-forming milk). That's why oranges are an essential nutritional tool in the treatment of bronchitis, sinusitis, tonsillitis, and sore throat. I regularly prescribe this citrus to combat common viral infections such as colds and the flu. A glass of fresh o.j. can prevent such nasty bugs.

Oranges are also good for the arteries. They keep cholesterol low and prevent plaque buildup in the blood vessels. Juice fasting, with an emphasis on fresh squeezed Valencia oranges, is extremely beneficial to blood pressure.

Nutrient Value: As mentioned above, the vitamin C and bioflavonoid content of this fruit make it a standout. The orange is also endowed with respectable levels of folic acid, vitamin B_1, and carotenoids. Its pectin content (see apples, below) has cholesterol-lowering value.

Selection and Care: The orange originated in southern China and Southeast Asia, and has become the leading fruit crop in the United States. I prefer thin-skinned California Valencia oranges for juicing, because they're sweeter and less sharp than other varieties. For eating, use thicker-skinned navels and Florida oranges. Tangerines and tangelos have similar personality traits to their sister citrus.

Select oranges that are heavy for their size. Avoid spongy, soft, puffy, or indented oranges. Surface scars and mottling are not important, so don't fret over these superficial flaws.

Optimal Use and Combining: Oranges are best used for juice or cut into segments as part of a fruit salad. They combine well with other citrus fruits, such as grapefruit or pineapple. Bananas and papayas also match up. But avoid mixing oranges with melons and other alkaline fruits. Citrus and melon are a poor food combo. And although oranges agree with strawberries in smoothies or fruit salads, they don't get along as well with apples, grapes, and other sub-acid fruits. For a gratifyingly crunchy snack, mix oranges with nuts, especially almonds, or with high-protein granola.

GRAPEFRUITS

Notable Personality Factors: Grapefruits—particularly the pink variety—are the ultimate emotional *adaptogen:* They lift deflated spirits and soothe anxious hyperactivity by balancing hormones and moods. They're glad foods. When you want to feel bright, right, and cheerful, grab a grapefruit. When you want to lose weight, down a glass of fresh squeezed grapefruit juice. Like oranges, grapefruits are a great way to start the day. Fit one into your Sunrise Cleanse, after your morning workout and right before you meditate.

Therapeutic and Healing Powers: I consider grapefruits to be the leading circulatory antiseptic. In other words, these power citruses are potent blood cleansers, which is precisely why they're so valuable in the prevention and treatment of bacterial and viral infections. Whenever you sense mucus accumulating in your throat or sinuses, or whenever you feel pressure in your ears, think grapefruits. They have excellent therapeutic value against colds, coughs, the flu, and bronchial or sinus infections. Use grapefruit and its rind to lower fevers and alleviate earaches.

Grapefruits are not only emotional but also physiological adaptogens: When the body needs to produce more red blood cells, grapefruits stimulate bone marrow. That's why they're a useful adjunct against anemia. Conversely, when the blood's red cell count and hemoglobin levels are too high, such as in a condition called polycythemia, grapefruits' adaptogenic properties decrease the excess production.

I prescribe grapefruits for any cardiovascular condition. In addition to cleansing the blood, they lower blood pressure, lower cholesterol levels with the aid of their pectin content, and prevent atherosclerosis and clotting. Grapefruits are a valuable component in a diet geared toward the prevention of Alzheimer's, senility, and stroke. In 300 B.C., the Greek philosopher and historian Theophrastus described the pulp of the grapefruit as the antidote to poison.

As with other citrus fruits, grapefruits are good for the immune system. They fight off cancer, and their high acid content enables them to break down and dissolve accumulated mucus in the glands, sinus, throat, or bronchial tubes.

Grapefruits also have a favorable influence on the metabolism. Anyone interested in permanent weight loss should be certain to have grapefruits and grapefruit juice as part of a daily diet. Both eliminate appetitis. If you're feeling ravenous, have a glass of fresh squeezed grapefruit juice mixed with one tablespoon of brewer's yeast and one tablespoon of spirulina or Revita—it will satisfy your hunger.

Nutrient Value: Grapefruits are rich in vitamins B_1 and C, flavonoids, and folic acid, and their water-soluble fiber has cholesterol-lowering properties.

Selection and Care: To ensure juiciness, choose grapefruits by weight rather than by size. Pick firm, thin-skinned, ripe grapefruits; avoid spongy, soft, indented ones. And note the ends of the grapefruit: When they are pointed, the fruit is likely to be thick-skinned and less juicy. The pink or red grapefruits have higher concentrations of vitamin A, enzymes, and fat-burning metabolites, so look for Ruby Red or Star Ruby from Florida or Texas crops.

Optimal Use and Combining: Eat grapefruits fresh, raw, and whole. Grapefruits combine well with other citrus, but don't mix well with alkaline melons or sub-acidic apples and berries. A salad of pink grapefruits with pineapples and bananas is my personal favorite in the winter and spring. Papayas also make excellent partners for pink grapefruits. Grapefruits invigorate nuts and granola, so make them a part of your trail mix when hiking or camping. And as part of a seasonal juice fast, emphasize fresh squeezed grapefruit and Valencia orange juices. Both are extremely beneficial to blood pressure.

PINEAPPLES

Notable Personality Factors: Native to South America and a staple of Hawaiian and other South Pacific cuisines, the pineapple has a playful effect on moods. It's a jubilant fruit, capable of creating upbeat, cheerful food swings. Like a tropical vacation, pineapples have a way of unwinding the body and mind.

Therapeutic and Healing Powers: Like all citrus fruits, pineapples cleanse the bloodstream, strengthen the immune system, and boost the metabolism. They, too, loosen up the mucus created by colds, the flu, and upper respiratory infections. But the pineapple's active ingredient—its secret weapon—is bromelain: This miracle phytonutrient, the protein-digesting enzyme complex of the fruit, resembles the enzymes in the sap of fig and papaya trees. I mention this because the same way sap heals a tree, so, too, does bromelain heal the body. In addition to treating indigestion and aiding in the breakdown of protein, bromelain has the notable ability to mend sports injuries and ease arthritic pain. In fact, bromelain is prescribed by plastic and general surgeons post-operatively, to reduce swelling of tissues and to prevent edema. It's used to inhibit blood platelet aggregation and accelerate wound healing. Because pineapple encourages an increase in hemoglobin, it is a valuable fruit for anyone suffering from anemia. Also, bromelain can be taken daily—instead of aspirin, as conventional cardiologists recommend—to prevent coronary or stroke.

Nutrient Value: In addition to bromelain, pineapples contain significant amounts of vitamins C and B_1.

Selection and Care: Fragrance is the key to determining freshness: A sweet aroma indicates that the fruit is mature. Look for bright green tops, securely attached crowns, and choose the deepest yellow-orange pineapples. Try to pull out one of the spines—if the pineapple is ripe, it will come out easily. The fruit should feel dry and heavy for its size, and should be free of dark, decayed spots.

Optimal Use and Combining: Serve pineapple fresh with other citrus fruits. Pineapple with strawberry and banana, pineapple with pink grapefruit and banana, or pineapple with papaya and banana all make excellent fruit salads. (However, pineapple does not combine well with melons or grapes.) Give granola a jolt with pineapple chunks.

SUB-ACID FRUITS

APPLES

Notable Personality Factors: The Granny Smith, the Macintosh, the Golden Delicious—there are more than twenty-five varieties of apples, and each has its own identity. But in general, apples are known for their take-charge personalities. They sharpen the mind, refresh the body, and strengthen resolve (just imagine the sort of determination Johnny Appleseed must have had to plant all those trees!). Apples revive confidence, cool down hot tempers, and generally encourage you to release tension and express feelings in order to regain emotional equilibrium.

Therapeutic and Healing Powers: We've all heard the expression "an apple a day keeps the doctor away." Since the ancient civilization of Greece, apples have been regarded as the antidote to many ailments, including those of the liver, gall bladder, nervous system, and skin. But the apple's most potent therapeutic benefit is it cardio-protective effect. It guards the heart from disease. Nutritionists credit this fantastic characteristic to the apple's pectin content. Pectin, found in the skin of the apple, is a remarkable fiber that has been proven to lower blood pressure and LDL, while increasing HDL (the bad and good cholesterols, respectively). In this way, it prevents arterial plaque from accumulating. Because pectin is a gel-forming fiber, it also increases the tone of the intestinal tract and promotes the elimination of toxic waste in the bowels and the bile. For this reason, apples are excellent for both the liver and for bowel regularity.

Fresh, whole apples and apple juice are high in chlorogenic, caffeic, and ellagic acid—cancer-fighting phytonutrients that have been shown to prevent tumors from forming. Interestingly, these phytonutrients are eliminated in canning or cooking processes—all the more reason to eat fruit fresh, alive, and raw.

Finally, if I still haven't sold you on the amazing apple, note that apples can decrease appetite and, thanks to their low glycemic index, slowly and steadily increase blood sugar. Apples also have antiviral properties and help to prevent colds and upper respiratory ailments such as bronchitis and laryngitis.

Nutrient Value: Along with their power triad of phytonutrients and their fibrous pectin, apples are high in potassium, vitamin A, and trace minerals.

Selection and Care: Back in the early 1990s, farmers used to spray apples with Alar, a chemical which caused apples to ripen uniformly. However, the pesticide was also a neurotoxin, and after the media caught on to the story, the Department of Consumer Affairs pulled the treated produce off the market and prohibited the use of the chemical. Considering the Alar publicity scare, it's advisable to buy organic apples, free of commercial waxes and pesticides, whenever possible. Fresh apples should be crisp, firm, and they should crunch when you bite them. Soft apples are not yet ripe, while spotted, brown, mushy ones are past their prime.

Optimal Use and Combining: Apples are an all-purpose fruit that enhance breakfast cereals, lunchtime salads, even desserts. They complement the flavors of pears, bananas, and papayas, but don't mix quite as well with citrus or melon.

BERRIES

Notable Personality Factors: Strawberries, blueberries, raspberries, currants—berries are colorful, popular fruits. Everybody looks forward to berry season, and with good reason. Berries bring a wonderful burst of flavor to fruit salads and smoothies. They're upbeat day-brighteners. The strawberry hails from Europe and the Americas, raspberries originated in the Middle East, and currants come from central Asia. Man has been relying on them for millennia. For example, physicians in Ancient Rome used strawberries to cure scurvy.

Therapeutic and Healing Powers: In spite of their small size, berries pack a therapeutic punch because of their high flavonoid content. Flavonoids are the plant pigments responsible for the fruits' coloration, and their chemistry protects them from environmental damage. Ingested, these flavonoids manifest into remarkable antioxidants. They protect against free radical damage and are anti-carcinogenic. Furthermore, the flavonoid content of berries prevents both the inflammation and degeneration of collagen and other connective tissues. By protecting small blood vessels and capillaries against leaking, berries act as an inter-cellular cement.

Anthocyanosides—flavonoids found in both the skin and substance of berries—potentiate the benefits of vitamin C, which, in turn, protects against the hardening of the arteries. The abundance of proanthocyanins, quercetin, 4-oxo-flavonoids, and other phytonutrients makes berries viricidal fruits that can be used to fight off infection. Blueberries help to treat diarrhea. Billberry prevents macular degeneration and the development of cataracts. Due to its ability to acidify urine, cranberry is commonly prescribed to treat bladder infections.

Nutrient Value: Berries are a very good source of vitamins B_1 and C. They are also high in vitamin E, potassium, water-soluble fiber, and antioxidants. Blueberries are high in manganese.

Selection and Care: Buy berries fresh, when they are in season. Select ripe, firm, well-shaped, brightly colored berries. Strawberries should be free of white or green tips, and raspberries should not show any blackening or mold. Avoid bruised or soft berries. Ideally, shop for organic berries, and use a biodegradable rinse on sprayed, non-organic brands.

Optimal Use and Combining: Berries mix well with other sub-acidic fruits, such as apples, peaches, cherries, and grapes. They also complement banana and papaya. Strawberry can hold its own with citrus, but, in general, berries don't match up as well with melons. Of course, berries add juicy flavor to nuts and granola. In summer, few foods are as refreshing as a strawberry smoothie.

GRAPES

Notable Personality Factors: Grapes have been associated with celebration for centuries, and today they are the leading fruit crop in the world. Why? Wine, of course. But even before they've been fermented, grapes can intoxicate. They're friendly, amorous fruits. In Caesar's Rome, grapes were kept on hand as aphrodisiacs.

Therapeutic and Healing Powers: Much has been made of the so-called "French paradox"—the generally good health of the French, in spite of the fact that their diet is high in red meat, butter, and cream. One of the suspected reasons behind this seeming contradiction has to do with the consumption of red wine. Grapes contain high concentrations of specific polyphenols and tannins. These act as antioxidizing agents and, as a result, have been linked to the prevention of cancer. The skin of grapes is high in fiber, and this is also part of the rationale behind the European view of grapes as cancer-curing agents.

Grape seed extract is rich in flavonoids and so, like other berries, grapes help to protect against the hardening of the arteries. Grape seed extract is also used to treat hemorrhoids, varicose veins, and phlebitis.

Grapes and grape juice have commonly been prescribed to cure viral infections, and for years nutritionists have recommended that patients go on an all-grape diet for seven to 10 days in order to thoroughly cleanse the blood and bowels.

Nutrient Value: Like other berries, grapes are high in flavonoids, potassium, trace minerals, and vitamin A.

Selection and Care: Grapes do not ripen after harvesting. Shake clusters well to dislodge damaged berries. Look for fruit that is colorful, firm, and wrinkle-free. For sweetness, I recommend Thompson seedless green grapes.

Optimal Use and Combining: Grapes enhance the flavor of peaches, pears, plums, berries, and nectarines. They don't fare as well with citrus, and tend to oversweeten bananas and other components of fruit salad. On their own, raisins and fresh grapes make energizing snacks and enliven granola, nuts, and cereals.

ALKALINE FRUITS

BANANAS

Notable Personality Factors: They call it mellow yellow. Bananas have a soothing influence. They settle you down and soften you up. Thought to have originated in the South Pacific and then migrated to India, the banana today has a number of different guises. There is, of course, the traditional yellow "Chiquita" banana, eaten raw and ripe, plus Jamaican and Mexican red-skinned varieties, and the popular plantain, which is eaten unripe and cooked in South America.

Therapeutic and Healing Powers: Bananas are the beneficiary of an intriguing nutritional combination: They are exceedingly high in potassium but blessedly low in sodium. This dietary duality makes the banana a valuable constituent in a high-performance food plan. Because of their alkalinity, bananas combat arthritic, digestive, and epidermal conditions.

Bananas also have specific, significant therapeutic value in the treatment of diarrhea. Bluntly put, they're the constipating fruit. Bananas ease an assortment of digestive disorders, such as gastritis and stomach ulcers. Researchers have discovered that the banana, particularly the plantain, strengthens the stomach lining. This protective coating shields against acid damage. And because of their pectin content, bananas, like apples, lower cholesterol. That's good for the arteries and the heart.

Mashed bananas are nourishing for those who need a bland or soft diet— for example, patients who have difficulty swallowing due to esophagitis or after oral surgery. Bananas can be used to quiet down diverticulitis, and athletes will be interested to learn that these wonder fruits, eaten alone or added to a smoothie, help to prevent muscle cramps.

Nutrient Value: Bananas are a solid source of potassium and vitamins A and B_1.

Selection and Care: Select golden yellow bananas flecked with brown spots. Green tips indicate that the fruit is not yet ripe. Store at room temperature until they ripen.

Optimal Use and Combining: Bananas are an alkaline fruit, but because they have such a mild taste and creamy texture, they combine well with apples, pears, pineapples, and papayas. Banana with pineapple and either strawberry or papaya makes a grounding morning fruit salad. A smoothie with fresh squeezed oranges, strawberries, and almonds works as a superb midday pick-me-up. Bananas are right at home in a bowl of granola, but, even though they are spreadable, because they are a starchy fruit, they are not the optimum choice for seven-grain toast.

CANTALOUPES

Notable Personality Factors: Cantaloupes are compassionate fruits, soulful, sensitive, and affectionate. They nurture the spirit, instill a sense of appreciation for life's gifts, and help to put priorities in proper order. Thought to have originated in Africa, cantaloupes are now grown all over the world.

Therapeutic and Healing Powers: Like citrus fruits, the alkaline cantaloupe cleanses and thins the blood. As such, it works to prevent platelet aggregation, which keeps blood from clotting. For this reason, cantaloupes make excellent components of a diet geared toward treating phlebitis and heart arrhythmia and preventing stroke. In addition to purifying the blood, cantaloupes also help clear out any sludge in the lymph system. Fresh squeezed cantaloupe juices purges toxins from the liver, spleen, and sinuses.

High in antioxidants, cantaloupes are considered to be anti-carcinogenic, and to specifically target breast and lung cancer. Like all alkaline fruits, cantaloupes also counteract liver stress. Finally, cantaloupes flush out the intestines and are excellent for elimination.

Nutrient Value: Nutrient-dense, high in vitamins A, B, and C, carotenes and other carotenoids, and unusually high in calcium, cantaloupes have a lot to offer a smart diet. They are particularly valuable for their heavy concentrations of B_3, folic acid, and pantothenic acid. Their potassium and magnesium contents contribute to their alkalinity.

Selection and Care: Choose firm cantaloupes with thick, rugged veining on the surface skin. When ripe, cantaloupes emit a sweet aroma.

Optimal Use and Combining: Cantaloupes complement other melons, such as watermelon and honeydew. Their juicy yet fibrous texture also mixes well with papayas. However, folklore has it that it is best to eat melons alone for peak absorption! As part of a liquid fast program, cantaloupe juice blended with watermelon, papaya, and almond butter makes a dynamic smoothie. In keeping with its season, emphasize cantaloupes in summer.

PEARS

Notable Personality Factors: Calm, cool, collected: Pears are a peace-bearing fruit. The Bosc, Anjou, and Bartlett all bestow a sense of serenity. The pear originated in the Mideast but is now grown in both North America and Europe. A tranquilizing effect is its distinguishing personality trait.

Therapeutic and Healing Powers: Packed with water-soluble fiber, particularly pectin, pears rally around the heart, fight off atherosclerosis, and lower LDL cholesterol. Furthermore, the high fiber content makes pears a useful nutritional tool to treat constipation, irritable bowel syndrome, and spastic colon.

Pear juice works as a diuretic to reduce water retention. It also clears up acne and other complexion problems. Alkaline fruits, pears promote healthy stomach and liver functions. Puréed like applesauce, pears aid in the treatment of digestive disorders, esophagitis, hiatal hernia, and acid indigestion. Because they help to stimulate peristalsis, pears are excellent for maintaining digestive hygiene when intestinal sluggishness or constipation is a problem.

Nutrient Value: Pears are high in fiber, potassium, trace minerals, and vitamin B_1.

Selection and Care: Evaluate pears the same way you do avocados: The flesh should yield ever so slightly to pressure. Unlike other fruits, pears can be picked when slightly green and allowed to ripen in a cool, dry, dark storage place. At full maturity, the center of the pear will be coarse-grained and gritty. For immediate consumption, choose perfect, unbruised specimens—soft, but not mushy. Pears are ripe when they are full-colored: Bosc pears turn from green to brown, Bartlett from green to yellow.

Optimal Use and Combining: Pears mix well with papayas and bananas, and also with apples, especially the Fuji variety. They do not pair as well with citrus or melons. Pears add a sweet, juicy crunch to seven-grain toast spread with nut butters.

WATERMELONS

Notable Personality Factors: When it comes to fruit, watermelon is one of the kings of the kingdom. It makes you feel potent and proud, and its juice gives an electric energy boost. Native to tropical Africa, watermelon grows well in warm climates, and, like the sun, it feeds a good mood and a positive mental attitude.

Therapeutic and Healing Powers: Watermelon's most significant clinical contributions are to the kidneys and bloodstream. As a diuretic, it helps to activate kidneys and eliminate salt, water, and toxins. Due to its high water content, it is very beneficial to purifying the bloodstream. Watermelon is also a dietary weapon in the ongoing war against high blood pressure. Another way it helps to enhance kidney function and, in turn, lower blood pressure, is by dilating small blood vessels and decreasing pressure in large ones. In fact, a three-to-five day all-watermelon diet is known to substantially lower blood pressure.

As a highly alkaline fruit, watermelon counters arthritis and other toxic acidic conditions that result from excess intake of meat proteins, dairy, eggs, artificial sweeteners, caffeine, and alcohol. Watermelon can also be used to treat kidney infections, bladder infections, prostates, and psoriasis.

Nutrient Value: With its concentration of carotenoids and vitamins A and C, watermelon is an efficient anti-aging antioxidant. It also contains significant quantities of calcium and iron.

Selection and Care: It can be difficult to determine a watermelon's ripeness, so it's useful to know a reputable fruit dealer in your neighborhood. Good watermelons are symmetrical in shape, and their underside should be slightly yellow, rather than pale green. Avoid soft spots at stem ends and flat, dry spots at blossom ends. The best way to test for freshness is to thump the side of a watermelon while you are holding it, then listen for a tympanic hollow sound. After cutting it down to size, cover sections in saran wrap and store watermelon in the refrigerator.

Optimal Use and Combining: Serve wedges of watermelon on their own, or with other fresh cuts of melon. Watermelon combines well with papaya and banana, but does not complement citrus fruits, apples, vegetables, or most grains (except for whole grain toast with nut butter). Watermelon juice, a powerful kidney cleanser, is the elemental drink of summer.

CHAPTER 15
VEGETABLE PERSONALITIES

Your mother knew what she was talking about when she told you to eat your vegetables. Potent, plant-based foods, vegetables are the key to a balanced nutritional program. In fact, the word "vegetable" comes from the Latin verb for "enliven." A wide variety of green, yellow, and red veggies are available at market. The following fifteen are among the most personable.

AVOCADOS

Notable Personality Factors: Although actually a fruit, the avocado is commonly classified—and prepared—as a vegetable. A shrewd food, the avocado is capable of harmonizing moods, and is one of the primary emoto-nutritional adaptogens. Avocados encourage artistic and creative self-expression. They have a sensual texture, and have been considered a dietary aphrodisiac for centuries. Rich in natural oils, the avocado keeps mind and body lubricated. Nicknamed the "alligator pear," and also known as *aguacate*, it is native to South and Central America. In the United States, it is produced primarily in southern California.

Therapeutic and Healing Powers: The high iron content of the avocado makes it an essential food for the blood. For example, avocados are helpful in the prevention and treatment of anemia. The avocado's copper content works in conjunction with the iron in order to insure that both minerals are properly utilized. Rich in protein and vegetable fat, avocados provide essential amino acids and substantial calories to fuel the system, and are the healthy choice for anyone who needs to gain weight: The average avocado weighs in with about 300 calories. Avocados energize overworked metabolisms, and are excellent restorative foods for post-operative or post-chemotherapy patients.

Nutrient Value: Avocados are high in protein and fat, but the fat content is predominantly unsaturated and provides essential oleic and linoleic acids to the brain cells and nerve tissues. Avocados are a reliable source of vitamins B_1, B_3, B_6, and E, and of potassium. In fact, the lovable aguacate has more than twice the potassium of a banana.

Selection and Care: To determine if an avocado has the ideal soft, smooth texture on the inside, it's necessary to evaluate the outside: Avocados tend to ripen first at the tips, but are thoroughly ripe when the central, thickest portion yields ever so slightly to pressure. Unripe avocados stored at room temperature will gradually ripen. Avoid aguacates with brown spots or blemishes. Once sliced, avocados quickly perish; wrap unused portions, pit and all, and refrigerate.

Optimal Use and Combining: Because the avocado has such a pleasingly mild flavor, it combines well with many foods. It accents leafy green garden vegetables, counterbalances the zing of tomato-onion salsa, and makes an excellent guacamole dip for celery and carrot sticks. A corn tortilla filled with fresh vegetables, sprouts, and avocado slices is a nutritious lunch. For even more protein, combine avocados with beans in a burrito or tostada. Their creamy, pliant texture has earned them the nickname "vegetable butter," and they can be used as a spread on toast or a baked potato.

ARTICHOKES

Notable Personality Factors: The character of the artichoke is best explained by its origin: The vegetable comes from the majestic

Mediterranean, primarily the south of Spain, France, and Italy. These three great cultures feed the artichoke, which symbolizes warmth, relaxation, and luxury like that which is found along the Côte d'Azur. With such an association, artichokes can't help but bring pleasure to any meal.

Therapeutic and Healing Powers: Folklore has it that the artichoke acts as a safety valve for the liver. Physicians in ancient Mediterranean cultures alleged that the beloved vegetable buffered the liver against the ill effects of alcohol, and recommended that it always accompany the consumption of red wine. Turns out they were right: In the 1970s, scientists discovered that the active ingredient in the artichoke was cynarin, a caffeylquinic acid. Cynarin has been shown to regulate the biliary "tree"—the network of ducts through which bile, after being excreted by the liver, flows into the gallbladder. Because artichokes have a positive influence on the movement of bile, they do, in fact, shelter the liver from stress, damage, and aging. The leaves and heart have the highest concentration of protective phytonutrients. Artichokes are also known to lower cholesterol levels.

Nutrient Value: Artichokes are high in a starchy carbohydrate called inulin, which is good for diabetics: Along with insulin, it helps to regulate blood sugar. Artichokes are also a solid source of calcium and iron.

Selection and Care: Layers of dark green leaves and bracts (scales) encircle the soft, juicy heart at the center of the vegetable. Look for consistently colored vegetables that have compact, tight-fitting bracts. The best way to prepare an artichoke is to steam it: The scales can then be plucked off and dipped into salsa, an eggless mayonnaise, or a soy spread.

Optimal Use and Combining: Since artichokes are a starchy vegetable, they do not go well with other starches, such as bread, rice, or potatoes. Instead, eat your steamed artichoke with vegetable soup and a fresh green salad.

ASPARAGUS

Notable Personality Factors: Due to its phallic configuration, the asparagus has long enjoyed a reputation as a libido-enhancing aphrodisiac. If you're interested in increasing your sex appeal, consider making asparagus spears a central component of your vegetable medley. And don't be alarmed by the strong odor asparagus adds to urine: The amino acid asparagine, which heightens sexual response, also produces a characteristic scent when excreted. But it is not harmful, and it quickly fades upon emission.

Therapeutic and Healing Powers: In addition to its usefulness as a dietary solution to sexual disinterest or dysfunction, asparagus also acts as a diuretic, and can relieve water retention. It is regarded as a gentle kidney cleanser. Asparagus reduces high blood pressure, increases the concentration of hemoglobin, and helps to prevent anemia. For these reasons, it is one of the more important vegetables for the circulatory system. Because asparagus is an alkaline vegetable, high in green chlorophyll and potassium, it helps to treat arthritis, rheumatism, and sciatica.

Nutrient Value: Asparagus is unique among vegetables for its high protein content. It is also remarkably high in B vitamins, folic acid, riboflavin, and potassium.

Selection and Care: Asparagus are dark green when mature. Choose stalks that are tender but firm, not brittle, woody, or pithy. Tips should be tightly closed. Steam asparagus spears until tender, and serve as an appetizer with dips or as part of a crudités plate.

Optimal Use and Combining: Asparagus flavors pasta and baked potatoes, and helps to make a mixed vegetable dish a complete protein meal.

BEETS

Notable Personality Factors: Bright burgundy-colored beets are highly nutritious root vegetables native to northern Europe. Although in America they've got a bit of a bad reputation—kids get excited about beets as much as they do about math tests—these vegetables are actually quite a shrewd food. Beet sugar supplies a fast but healthy energy high, and is quickly burned as fuel. Beet fans find the vegetable invigorating and uplifting.

Therapeutic and Healing Powers: Beets are the liver's buddies. They reduce liver stress, clearing out sludge and sediment in the liver bed and bile. Because of this, they have an anti-depressant effect on the brain. Due to their alkalinity, beets also cleanse the bloodstream and kidneys. Their plentiful supply of phytonutrients are thought to contain anti-carcinogenic qualities. They can also be used to stimulate appetite.

Nutrient Value: Beets are high in potassium and trace minerals, while beet greens contain significant amounts of calcium, iron, folic acid, and vitamin A.

Selection and Care: Judge a beet by the freshness of its greens. Choose young roots with upright, frondlike tops, and look for purple-red beets that are firm, symmetrically shaped, and smooth. Avoid soft, dull-colored beets. Scrub beets well, and shred or pare the thin outer skin before cooking.

Optimal Use and Combining: Beets add a hearty snap to leafy green salads, and, from an aesthetic perspective, a pleasing punch of color to mixed vegetable plates—combined with pale green celery and vivid orange carrots, for example. From a therapeutic point of view, beets are most effective in fresh vegetable juices: Carrot-celery-beet juice really cleans out the liver. Steamed beets make an excellent dinner side dish, served alongside potatoes or brown rice. They can also be puréed into a borscht.

BROCCOLI

Notable Personality Factors: Forget about what former President Bush said. Broccoli rules! This nutrient-dense vegetable activates the brain, enlivens the nervous system, and bolsters the adrenals. That's why I refer to it as the ultimate "ready food." Broccoli sees to it that the body is prepared to deal with whatever physical or mental demands are at hand. It protects against stress, and promotes self-confidence. Italians can claim the credit for cultivating a farming technique that turned cabbage into broccoli.

Therapeutic and Healing Powers: As a member of the cruciferous, or cabbage, family (which also includes Brussels sprouts, cauliflower, kale, mustard greens, rutabagas, and turnips), broccoli is endowed with incredible cancer-inhibiting properties. Potent antioxidant phytonutrients such as indoles, glucosinolates, and dithiolthiones work hard to prevent cancer— particularly estrogen-related cancers—from developing. A highly alkaline green vegetable, broccoli is also good for the liver, kidneys, and spleen. Its high iron content benefits the blood. Steamed broccoli helps to boost the adrenal glands and alleviate fatigue. Its energizing capacity also counters depression and metabolic burnout.

Nutrient Value: Broccoli is blessed with mucho vitamins and minerals— calcium, folic acid, potassium—along with antioxidants, enzymes, and protein. In fact, there is more protein in a broccoli dinner than there is in bread or wheat. And it's low in calories. It gets its adrenal-building powers from its stock of pantothenic acid.

Selection and Care: Choose dark green broccoli. Buds should be tightly closed. Florets that have begun to soften and yellow are no longer ripe. Look for fresh green leaves and firm stalks. Broccoli can be steamed or enjoyed raw.

Optimal Use and Combining: Eat broccoli four to five times a week. It goes well with any vegetarian platter, and adds a wonderful crunch to pasta primavera. Broccoli makes a tasty partner for a baked potato.

CABBAGE

Notable Personality Factors: Cabbage is not quite as popular as its cruciferous sister, broccoli, which is a shame, because it can be quite revitalizing. Cabbage boosts the immune system. I consider it a "longevity food." Austria, Germany, and the countries of northern Europe and the former Soviet Union are major cabbage cultivators, preserving it for the winter months in the form of sauerkraut.

Therapeutic and Healing Powers: Like all other cruciferous veggies, cabbage combats cancer. Even the American Cancer Society says so. Fighter phytonutrients such as indoles and isothiocyanites block cancerous cell formation. Cabbages have been specifically linked to a lower incidence of colon cancer: The vegetable triggers the detoxification and elimination of harmful chemicals and hormones found in food, water, and air pollutants. Red cabbage regenerates the bowels, and green cabbage has been shown to successfully treat peptic ulcer disease. The vegetable's waste-removing abilities also benefit the liver.

Nutrient Value: All members of the cruciferous family are high in anticancer nutrients: flavonoids, indoles, phenols, and other antioxidants. Cabbages also contain a plentiful supply of vitamins C and E, calcium, iron, potassium, and fiber.

Selection and Care: Select fresh, firm, crisp cabbages with compact heads, heavy for their size, and tightly wrapped leaves free of discoloration at the edges.

Optimal Use and Combining: Raw green and red cabbage can be tossed in salads or grated for a vegan coleslaw. Cabbage soup is particularly fortifying in cold winter months. Cabbage, cauliflower, and the rest of the cruciferous family mix well with beets, carrots, and other root vegetables. Cabbage also adds a pungent flavor to vegetable soups, brown rice, and whole grain pasta.

CARROTS

Notable Personality Factors: Carrots energize and animate—where do you think Bugs Bunny gets all that get-up-and-gumption? A glass of fresh-squeezed carrot juice provides an almost-instant boost. Hundreds of years ago, carrots were used to treat nervous conditions. In their early incarnation, these root vegetables were, in fact, purple-black in color, but crop rotation in the Middle East eventually resulted in the characteristic orange flesh. Carrots are considered custodial foods. They shelter the systems from illness.

Therapeutic and Healing Powers: Carrots are another anti-cancer vegetable: Their beta-carotene content has been shown to prevent lung cancer and other smoking-related cancers, such as those of the throat, larynx, pancreas, and bladder. Reformed smokers who want to take preventive measures to insure against the late onset of such cancers would do well to eat two carrots a day. They are also beneficial to the prevention of other upper respiratory infections and inflammatory lung problems. Carrot, carrot-celery, and carrot-celery-beet juice are all excellent liver tonics, and the crunchy root vegetable also cleans the blood and regulates the bowels. Steamed carrots can be prescribed to treat diarrhea. By regenerating the thyroid and adrenal glands, carrots also combat metabolic burnout.

Nutrient Value: Carrots are a top source of vitamins A and B, rich in beta-carotene and other carotenoids, and high in calcium and potassium.

Selection and Care: Select firm, smooth roots. Avoid carrots that are rubbery, wrinkled, pithed, or split. Carrot greens should be bright and upright.

Optimal Use and Combining: Combine fresh carrots with cruciferous vegetables for an anti-cancer crudités plate. Carrot sticks make edible utensils for vegan mayonnaise, almond butter spreads, tomato-onion salsa, and fresh guacamole. Chopped raw carrots add crunch to leafy green salads and mix especially well with zucchini and romaine lettuce. Steamed carrots make a tasty side for a baked potato. Refrigerate carrots prior to blending them into juice, and if the taste of fresh carrot juice seems a little strong for the untrained stomach, sweeten the drink with a touch of apple.

CUCUMBERS

Notable Personality Factors: Even though it hails from the tropics, the cuke is the king of cool. Its juicy, soothing flesh calms overheated nerves. In summer, cucumbers' mild flavor refreshes salads.

Therapeutic and Healing Powers: Cucumbers have a high water content and therefore help to flush unwanted toxins out of the systems, regulate bodily fluids, and cleanse blood. The skin of the cucumber contains silica, a mineral essential to the growth of connective tissue and skin.

Nutrient Value: Cucumbers contain erepsin, an enzyme that improves protein digestion. They're also a low-calorie vegetable high in vitamin B_1 as well as minerals and trace elements.

Selection and Care: Cucumbers should be firm and consistently colored, with medium to dark green, unwaxed skin. Young, fresh cukes can be eaten skin and all, but if the skin is tough, pare the vegetable to avoid digestive disruptions. Shriveling and yellowness are signs that a cucumber is past its prime. And, since they are heavily salted, pickled cucumbers should be considered an occasional indulgence.

Optimal Use and Combining: Raw cucumber with watercress and jicama makes a refreshing spring or summer salad.

GARLIC

Notable Personality Factors: Garlic's reputation as a miracle cure goes back to antiquity. Bulbs decorated the walls of Egyptian tombs dating from 3000 B.C., presumably as part of some religious ritual. Hippocrates and Plato praised garlic for its medicinal properties. Folklore refers to it as the remedy for warding off everything from parasitic infections to vampire attacks. Today, garlic is grown worldwide, and used to season all sorts of dishes.

Therapeutic and Healing Powers: More so than with almost any other vegetable, it's tough to separate fact from fiction when it comes to defining garlic's therapeutic properties. In general, dieticians agree that garlic's nutritional benefits fall into three categories:

Cardiovascular: Two to three cloves of garlic a day helps to lower total cholesterol while elevating good, HDL, cholesterol. This, in turn, helps to prevent hardening of the arteries. Garlic is also reputed to thin the blood and prevent the formation of clots. It naturally lowers blood pressure. Considering its cholesterol-lowering, anti-clotting, anti-hypertensive effects, garlic is good for the heart.

Anti-infectious: Garlic has been called "Russian penicillin," and the Japanese have popularized kyolic, a liquid extract of cold-processed garlic, as a treatment for bacteria and viruses. It has also been used to cure candida, various fungi, and parasitic worms. Garlic's antibiotic properties help to fortify the immune system and defend against infections.

Anti-cancerous: Laboratory experiments have documented garlic's ability to kill cancer cells through its stimulant effect on the immune system.

Nutrient Value: Garlic is rich in enzymes, trace minerals, germanium, selenium, and sulfur-containing allicin (the element responsible for garlic's sharp odor).

Selection and Care: Look for firm bulbs with tightly packed cloves encased in thin, papery skin. Avoid garlic that has begun to sprout, or that is graying, soft, and decaying in spots.

Optimal Use and Combining: Roasted garlic adds flavor to almost anything: mashed potatoes, pasta, soups. It can even be used as a spread on whole wheat bread.

LETTUCE

Notable Personality Factors: Like garlic, lettuce also has a centuries-old reputation as a healer. Lettuce originated in the Mediterranean, and at various times Greek, Roman, and French physicians prescribed it for medicinal purposes. Caesar credited the leafy vegetable with his recovery from various ailments. Lettuce lovers swear by the benefits of its vitamins, minerals, and nutrients, and turn to the vegetable for its tranquilizing effect. I believe romaine lettuce is superior to other types of lettuce. Specifically, the darker the leaf, the greater the nutritional value. That's why bitter greens such as arugula and spinach also make a powerful dietary impact, while milder forms of lettuce, such as butterhead or iceberg, are less nutritious. Romaine is also renowned for its aphrodisiacal effects.

Therapeutic and Healing Powers: Due to its high concentration of chlorophyll, romaine lettuce is invaluable to the prevention of disease. It is a central aid in waste elimination, it cleanses the liver, and it protects against cancers of the colon, rectum, and intestines. Romaine salads boost the immune system, bolster the blood, and prevent anemia, the flu, and other infections.

Nutrient Value: In addition to being packed with powerful chlorophyll, romaine lettuce contains an incredible arrangement of B-complex vitamins and essential trace minerals.

Selection and Care: Prime romaine lettuce is crisp, leafy, and firm. It stands up straight. Examine the head for wilted leaves or rotting, discolored edges, both of which are signs of spoilage. The average-sized head of lettuce yields four large salad servings. Wash lettuce well by removing and rinsing one leaf at a time with cool water, and store unused portions in the refrigerator.

Optimal Use and Combining: Romaine is the basis for any green salad. It mixes well with other lettuces for a mesclun salad, and with yellow, orange, and red veggies for a crunchy tossed salad. The heart of romaine lettuce is the key component of Caesar salad.

MUSHROOMS

Notable Personality Factors: Long considered an ornamental food, mushrooms such as the reishi and shiitake actually have incredible energizing powers. The ancient cultures of China valued mushrooms as longevity-promoting vegetables. Psychedelic mushrooms grow wild in Central and South America, as well as in the southwestern United States, and their mind-altering properties probably earned them their reputation as a spiritual, medicinal food. Mushrooms are also associated with sensuality and sexuality. Because they are a fungus, they should be avoided by anyone suffering from candida or yeast infections. Even though different types of mushrooms sprout openly in all sorts of climates, some varieties are poisonous, and amateurs should not attempt to distinguish the good from the bad. Instead, buy mushrooms from any reputable market.

Therapeutic and Healing Powers: Reishi and shiitake mushrooms boost the immune system by producing interferon-like effects that fight viral infection. Mushrooms are also being studied for their anti-cancerous capabilities. The button mushroom, popular in the United States, is loaded with enzymes which aid the digestive process. For this reason, they are useful dietary tools for elderly patients suffering from indigestion. The popular portobello mushroom, also high in protein, makes an aromatic garnish for tofu and vegetable dishes.

Nutrient Value: Mushrooms are rich in potassium, copper, iron, and other essential minerals and proteins. They contain a valuable sulfurous amino acid, methionine, and are an excellent source of vitamin B_1. For a vegetable, they have a high fat content (8%), and their alkalinity contributes to liver vitality and blood chemistry.

Selection and Care: Mushrooms are sold as "buttons," with closed heads attached to their stem, or "open caps," fanned out and cut from their stem. Button mushrooms should be firm, bulbous, and white. Other varieties, such as the portobello mushroom, will range in color from golden to gray-brown on the topside, and dark brown to nearly black on the underside. Mushrooms have a naturally velvety texture, but keep an eye out for rotting spots. Wash mushrooms under running water, and use a soft brush to remove condensed dirt from the rounded cap.

Optimal Use and Combining: Mushrooms can be steamed, baked, boiled, fried, grilled, or sautéed, but prolonged cooking removes their flavor, making them bland and rubbery. Tossed raw in a leafy green salad, they retain their dense, slightly nutty taste. Combined with tofu, mushrooms make a complete protein. They also accent brown rice, pasta, and steamed green vegetables, and add texture to a chunky marinara sauce.

ONIONS

Notable Personality Factors: Due to their pungent odor, sharp taste, and tear-inducing ability, onions are the cause of much controversy. It's a love-hate thing: There are those who admire the onion for its strength, and those who despise it for the exact same reason. Onions originated in central Asia and migrated to the Mideast. Today, a wide variety of onions are grown the world over. Like its fellow bulbous herb, garlic, the onion is alleged to cure many illnesses. Onions are an acidic vegetable; their organic sulfur compounds are responsible for stimulating the tear ducts.

Therapeutic and Healing Powers: Onions are reputed to lower cholesterol, blood sugar, and blood pressure. By extension, they are considered a natural antibiotic. Their sharp, spicy taste tends to clear out the sinuses, and onion-based soup has long been considered a folk remedy for sore throats, tonsillitis, and the common cold. Raw onion relaxes the bronchial muscles, which makes it a useful food in the treatment of asthma. Because onions increase the effectiveness of insulin, they are also viable dietary aids for diabetics. Some researchers have attributed anti-cancer properties to raw onions; others regard them as a sleep aid.

Nutrient Value: Onions are a good source of vitamins B_1 and C, calcium, sodium, and sulfur.

Selection and Care: Soft, damp onions are usually spoiled, and have lost their flavor. Choose firm bulbs, yellow-, green-, or red-skinned, according to personal preference (although red onions are less acidic than other varieties). When preparing onions, peel the outermost layers under cold running water: This will help to prevent crying in the kitchen.

Optimal Use and Combining: Mild onions are best eaten raw, minced or sliced in salads or sandwiches. Stronger varieties can be baked, boiled, broiled, or steamed. Onions are essentially a seasoning, and can be used in small quantities to flavor vegetarian entrees and tomato salsas and sauces. Never salt onions—they're naturally high in sodium.

POTATOES

Notable Personality Factors: Potatoes are a versatile, popular, staple starch. Native to the South American Andes, somewhere between Bolivia and Peru, the potato made its way to Europe via the Spanish explorers, and, of course, found a second home in Ireland. Potatoes have a grounding effect on the digestive system, and help the stomach to feel sated. They hit the spot on cold, rainy days. They're comfort food—but they also fuel the metabolism.

Therapeutic and Healing Powers: Because of their high glycemic index, potato nutrients are rapidly absorbed and swiftly raise blood sugar. Although potatoes are a member of the nightshade family, which has a reputation for causing arthritis, I believe that, as highly alkaline vegetables, potatoes are beneficial for rheumatism, sciatica, and other musculo-skeletal disorders. The only obvious exception would be for those who may have developed an allergy to nightshades: In their case, eating potatoes will worsen arthritis, and elimination of potatoes from the diet will result in an improvement of symptoms within three to five days.

Baked, potatoes are an excellent source of instant energy. They also treat such digestive disorders as spastic colon, diverticulitis, and ulcer disease. The mild taste and soft texture of potatoes makes them a good food for infants and the elderly. Contrary to their commercial, French-fried reputation, potatoes actually stimulate the metabolism to burn fat, and are elemental to permanent weight loss. A baked potato at dinner balances out an abundance of garden green vegetables.

Nutrient Value: Potatoes are an excellent source of vitamin C, minerals, potassium and, in particular, protein.

Selection and Care: Choose dry, firm, smooth-skinned, shallow-eyed potatoes with minimal blemishes. Green spots indicate sunburn, and will have a bitter taste, while deep pits and sprouting eyes are signs that the potato is past its prime. A uniformly round or elliptical shape helps to expedite the cooking process. Store potatoes in a paper bag in a dark, cool, well-ventilated spot.

Optimal Use and Combining: Baked potatoes are easier on the digestive system than hard-boiled potatoes, but the latter can be used in an eggless vegetarian potato salad. Potatoes ground green vegetables and work especially well with cauliflower and the Indian delicacy called *Aloo Gobi.* To season baked potatoes, use tomato salsa or avocado guacamole instead of butter and salt.

SPINACH

Notable Personality Factors: Spinach animates, invigorates, and energizes. It's a quick food. A call to action. Remember Popeye's relationship with the potent leaf? Pow! That's the spinach personality profile. Spinach is thought to have originated in Persia, and it's long been considered a medicinal vegetable.

Therapeutic and Healing Powers: Like other dark green lettuces, spinach is rich in chlorophyll. It's also endowed with the highest iron concentration of all its leafy relatives. This combination of chlorophyll and iron puts spinach in a class by itself. It builds the blood, strengthens the immune system, and nourishes bone marrow. Furthermore, spinach's peak phytonutrient content and anti-cancer antioxidants protect the liver and kidneys, and aid in the prevention of lung, stomach, colon, rectum, and prostate cancers.

Nutrient Value: In addition to its high iron and chlorophyll concentrations, spinach contains substantial quantities of vitamin A and B-carotenoids, copper, and potassium. However, spinach is not recommended for those with a history of kidney stones, since the vegetable's high oxalic acid concentration can contribute to stone formation.

Selection and Care: Spinach spoils quickly: Select leaves based on their crispness and brilliant emerald green color. Avoid coarse, wilted, limp, or yellow leaves, or those with blackening edges. Spinach shrinks significantly when cooked, so what seems like a large amount usually isn't. For example, a pound will yield three generous servings. Buy accordingly. Store spinach in tight containers in the fridge. Do not wash until ready to use.

Optimal Use and Combining: Spinach is most nutritious when eaten raw, mixed with chopped mushrooms, carrots, and zucchini as part of a tossed salad. But it can also be steamed. Spinach casseroles and spinach-seasoned tofu lasagna make hearty, healthy meals. The steamed leaves can also accent pasta, brown rice, or lentils, and they make a pungent partner for a baked potato.

TOMATOES

Notable Personality Factors: These bright red "passion fruits," dubbed "love apples" by the French, were once thought to be toxic. Native to South America, today the tomato is one of the world's leading vegetable crops. Tomatoes build the blood and boost brain power. Their invigorating chemistry sharpens discriminatory and analytical abilities. They clear the mind. They also clean the bowels. During the seventeenth and eighteenth centuries, physicians prescribed tomatoes as a preventive measure against appendicitis. Their juicy texture and vividly colored flesh contributes to their reputation as an aphrodisiac.

Therapeutic and Healing Powers: Tomatoes are chiefly blood builders and cleansers. As one of the more acidic vegetables—some authorities classify them as a fruit—they clear mucus from upper respiratory passages. For this reason, tomatoes help to cure the common cold, the flu, bronchitis, and sinus infections. They also burn away plaque from arteries and blood vessels. In recent years, medical literature has expounded on the plethora of high-density phytonutrients found in tomatoes. One theory holds that tomatoes can counter lung and stomach cancers: Their lycopene content has been credited with the prevention of prostate cancer. Tomatoes also help to regulate peristalsis and to eliminate fecal toxins.

Nutrient Value: Red tomatoes are high in vitamin C, B-carotene and other carotenoids, such as lycopene. A medium-sized tomato has one-and-a-half grams of fiber.

Selection and Care: Select tomatoes on the basis of color: They are ripe when bright red, tight-skinned, and firm to the touch. Avoid split or bruised flesh.

Optimal Use and Combining: Fresh raw tomatoes juice up leafy green salads. Combined with onions, they make a chunky, tangy salsa or spaghetti sauce. Although there are some popular canned tomato juices on the market, carrot juice is a more alkaline vegetable juice option.

CHAPTER 16
GRAIN PERSONALITIES

Grains, most commonly in the forms of bread and rice, are staple foods that have fed most of the world's population for millennia—wheat and barley date back some 10,000 years. Today, with the increasing birthrate and subsequent demands on agriculture, grains are as important as ever.

Because they're high in complex carbohydrates, dietary fiber, vitamins, minerals, enzymes, and amino acids, grains are also essential components of a high-performance nutrition plan. To provide complete proteins, grains are best matched with legumes—brown rice with beans, for example. Bread, cereal, rice, and pasta made from whole grains are superior to their processed, white-flour counterparts.

PREPARING WHOLE GRAINS

When cooking grains, use a pot or saucepan with a tight-fitting lid. Bring water to a boil and slowly stir in grain. Simmer, covered, for as long as recommended, depending on the quantity: Pots and pans vary, so a certain amount of trial and error is inevitable, and the times listed below are approximations. Do not stir during the simmer stage. All water should be absorbed by the grain once it is cooked, but eliminate any residual moisture by draining the grains in a colander. Fluff lightly with a fork before serving.

COOKING TIME FOR GRAINS		
GRAIN (1 cup dry)	WATER	TIME
barley, pearl	2½ cups	1 hour
buckwheat groats, raw	3 cups	20–25 minutes
cornmeal and corn grits	4 cups	30 minutes
millet	3 cups	30 minutes
oats, whole	3 cups	1 hour
oats, flaked or rolled	3 cups	30 minutes
rice, brown, short-grain	2 cups	50 minutes
rice, brown, long-grain	2 cups	40–50 minutes
rye berries	2½ cups	1 hour
rye flakes	2 cups	20 minutes
wheat berries	2½ cups	1 hour
wheat bulgur	2 cups	15–20 minutes
wheat flakes	2 cups	20 minutes

Although there are some 5,000 varieties of grains, the following three are the most popular and prevalent:

WHEAT

Notable Personality Factors: Wheat is the most popular grain in the world, a dietary staple of more than one-third of the earth's population—hence its description as "the staff of life." Artifacts dating back 10,000 years indicate that ancient Egyptians farmed the grain on the Fertile Crescent.

Due to its gluten content, wheat is considered the best grain for bread-baking. Although gluten is found in other grains as well, it has its highest concentration in wheat. Comprised of two allergenic proteins, gluten causes bread to rise.

Whether it's toast with cereal for breakfast, sandwiches with soup for lunch, or a loaf to accompany dinner, whether it's a New York bagel, a French baguette, Belgian waffles, or Indian nan, bread is considered indispensable to almost any meal in almost every culture. "Breaking bread" refers to the communal aspect of the grain: Sharing it symbolizes friendship and affection. But for many, bread has become a comfort food that takes the place of true emotional nutrition. Excess consumption can wreak havoc on the metabolism, and those who are overweight or suffering from thyroid dysfunctions should seriously consider eliminating it from their diets. Moreover, an allergic reaction to wheat is often the cause behind such chronic digestive dysfunctions as colitis, indigestion, diarrhea, and malabsorption syndrome. Although it usually affects the digestive tract, wheat allergy can also, in rare instances, result in recurrent bronchitis or recurrent bladder infections. Those afflicted with autoimmune disorders should eliminate wheat from their diets for at least six weeks.

Therapeutic and Healing Powers: A high-fiber food, whole wheat protects the digestive tract, liver, and colon. Because it nourishes the central nervous system, wheat is also considered brain food, and it has a grounding effect on anxiety and erratic emotions. By extension, it provides energy, particularly for tasks that demand stamina and endurance—in other words, long-distance running as opposed to jackrabbit sprints! As a fiber supplement, one to two tablespoons of miller's bran is a powerful bowel regulator and helps the body properly form and eliminate stools.

Nutrient Value: Whole wheat contains much more protein than refined wheat flour. It's rich in B vitamins, protein, zinc, pantothenic acid, magnesium, chromium, other trace minerals, and essential fatty acids. It's also high in antioxidants.

Selection and Care: Choose whole wheat over refined white bread, and store in a paper bag inside a bread tin, so that the bread can breathe. Breads do not have a very long shelf life—keep an eye out for the development of mold. However, dried organic cereals and bran powders can be stored for quite a while: Just be sure to close the containers tightly.

Optimal Use and Combining: Build sandwiches—avocado, hommus, vegetarian burgers—on whole wheat breads, buns, and pita pockets. A slice of toast spread with almond butter can be served alongside vegetable soup. Or add bran powders to fruit smoothies for fiber.

RICE

Notable Personality Factors: According to legend, the Buddha could eat a bowl of rice one kernel at a time. To slowly chew on each individual grain was a form of meditation. Students of Zen, mirroring the master, aim to chew each kernel until they feel the water content of the rice released through their careful mastication. This teaches the value of food. The point is, you can eat the same bowl of rice in mere minutes or a full hour: How you choose to respect your food is up to you.

Rice is a balancing, yin-yang grain that acts as a powerful metabolic cleanser. On the yin side, it's a serene, nurturing food. On the yang, it replenishes energy. Macrobiotic nutrition emphasizes the healing characteristics of rice, but note that, although processed, boil-in-a-bag white rice may be more readily available, long grain, basmati, and brown rice are all healthier alternatives.

Therapeutic and Healing Powers: Rice is the go-to grain for digestive disturbances. Colitis, esophagitis, intestinal flu, ulcers, and upset stomachs all respond positively to rice. It's easy to digest and assimilate, but because it's high in fiber, it also cleans out the intestinal tract. Rice-based cereals are particularly helpful in combating diarrhea, diverticulitis, constipation, and other symptoms of an irritable bowel. And rice nurtures the liver and pancreas, two organs crucial to carbohydrate metabolism.

When it's necessary to eliminate wheat grains from the diet due to indigestion or gluten allergy, rice noodles are the ideal substitute. When there's a combination of wheat and dairy allergies, as is often the case with colitis and recurrent bronchial or bladder infections, rice is all the more important. Rice noodles, brown rice cakes, and rice-based crackers fit into a no-wheat plan—and help to correct the functional hypoglycemia and stabilize the excessive weight loss that may accompany stomach or colon disorders.

For infants three to six months old, rice cereal is a good starter solid. Rice milk and cheese are also nutritious alternatives to cow's milk and pasteurized cheeses. Rice can calm down and open up driven Type-A personality types. A combination of rice, tofu, and green vegetables provides complete proteins and total nutrition.

Nutrient Value: Rice has a higher quality to its protein than wheat. Its chief nutritional components are fiber, minerals, and B vitamins.

Selection and Care: Rice is sold dried, and can be stored indefinitely. Select brown, basmati, and whole grain varieties over refined white rice. Avoid prepackaged, powdered sauces, and flavor instead with natural herbs and spices.

Optimal Use and Combining: Brown rice can ground almost any meal: a leafy green salad, a tempeh dinner dish, a vegetarian paella. Mix with beans for proteins and add dense, crunchy vegetables like broccoli, mushroom, and asparagus for flavor. For a snack, spread rice cakes with guacamole, salsa, hommus, or almond butter.

CORN

Notable Personality Factors: Corn on the cob, corn tortillas, corn chips—not to mention that movie treat, popcorn—are all popular American foods. In fact, they've come to evoke the feeling of the Fourth of July or the county fair. While corn does not have the nutritional potency of wheat or rice, it still benefits the body in many ways, and should be included in a high-performance diet as an adjunct grain.

Therapeutic and Healing Powers: Cornmeal and corn tortillas aid the digestive system, although the whole kernels of corn on the cob are harder to digest than, for example, rice, and so may not belong in the diets of those suffering from diverticulitis or other digestive problems. An energizing grain, corn protects the liver from stress and helps it to detoxify. Its high fiber content promotes regular elimination, which reduces the risk of cancer of the colon. Quesadillas made from corn tortillas with soy or rennetless cheese, or nachos of corn chips and the same soy or rice cheeses, both stimulate the glandular systems, and as such are excellent additions to the diets of women who are pregnant, women who are lactating, children, or those trying to gain weight. Burritos made from corn tortillas stuffed with guacamole and vegetables are a potent nutritional combo. Corn and beans also provide a complete protein.

Nutrient Value: Corn is a solid source of B vitamins, minerals, complex carbohydrates, and dietary fiber. When preparing tortillas or polenta, keep in mind that cornmeal ground with water and lime (a Mexican tradition) is particularly nutritious because the lime activates and releases the niacin (vitamin B_3) in the corn protein. Corn oil is high in polyunsaturated fat.

Selection and Care: In summer months, enjoy sweet corn on the cob. Look for firm, evenly colored husks and check the soft, hairlike strands at the top for any darkness or rotting. Buy organic corn chips and tortilla shells.

Optimal Use and Combining: After stripping away the outer leaves, boil corn on the cob for about seven minutes. To season, use avocado or salsa instead of butter and salt. These seasonings can also be used as dips for corn chips. For a substantial lunch or dinner, stuff corn tortillas with avocado, steamed vegetables, baked black or red beans, or rennetless or soy cheese.

While wheat, rice, and corn are the three most prominent and most popular grains, there are several others that can add variety to a high-performance nutritional program. Like the three main grains, all ground and calm. Consider incorporating the following into your meal plan:

Amaranth: An ancient Central American grain, amaranth is less allergenic than wheat and can take its place in breads or breakfast cereals. Something of a specialty food item, amaranth is more expensive than common grains.

Buckwheat: One of the few alkaline grains, buckwheat is a therapeutic choice for those afflicted with liver stress or other over-acidic conditions. For example, buckwheat pancakes make an excellent alkaline breakfast treat.

Kamut: A light, alkaline grain, kamut, like amaranth, can also be used as a wheat substitute in bread products (such as yeast-free kamut bagels).

Millet: Another highly alkaline grain, millet is light and easy to digest, and can be used as an alternative to both wheat and rice. Millet also has a higher grade of protein than other grains, making millet burgers very nutritious. Puffed millet with fruit and soy milk is a cleansing children's cereal.

Oats: Oat bran is known for its cholesterol-lowering effect. High-fiber, whole-grain oatmeal served with rice, soy, or almond-sesame milk makes a healthy breakfast cereal.

Quinoa: Primarily used as a wheat substitute, quinoa is even less allergenic than amaranth. A convenient grain, it cooks in about 20 minutes.

Triticale: A hybrid of wheat and rye, triticale contains more protein than either one of its individual constituents.

CHAPTER 17

LEGUME PERSONALITIES

For protein, nothing beats beans. High-fiber, low-fat, high-protein legumes are in a class by themselves. Due to their amazing ability to provide protein without the saturated fat that usually accompanies it in animal byproducts, legumes make an excellent substitute for meat and dairy. In fact, the protein in legumes is of a higher overall biological quality than the protein in animal byproducts: It does not damage key organs, as meat has been shown to do, and it is easier to digest and assimilate.

Legumes provide more protein than do fruits, vegetables, or grains, but for balanced meals, they are best combined with these items. Grains are low in lysine while legumes are high in the amino acid, for example, and legumes benefit from the methionine boost they get from mushrooms and grains.

MAGIC BEANS

What can't legumes do?

By promoting thorough detoxification, they reduce liver stress. By penetrating and accelerating the body's processing of carbohydrates, they relieve pancreatic stress. By regulating blood sugar, they aid in the prevention of diabetes. Their alkalinity makes legumes a nutritional ally of the kidneys—their uncanny ability to bind acids and acid toxins takes some of the pressure off the organs to do the same. The considerable fiber content in legumes helps to combat the growth of cancerous cells—soybeans, for example, have been linked to the prevention of breast cancer. In addition to their energy-boosting protein punch, legumes are endowed with an assortment of minerals and amino acids that calm the central nervous system: Combined with their phytonutrients, these two elements have also earned legumes their reputation as a dietary antidepressant. And legumes lower cholesterol, making them an invaluable weapon in the battle against metabolic enemy number one, hardening of the arteries. Anyone interested in lowering cholesterol naturally, without pharmaceuticals, would be wise to adopt a vegan diet of fruits, vegetables, grains, and legumes.

Compared to the immediate sweetness of fruits or the savory snap of vegetables, legumes have a more subtle, textured flavor. The thick, hearty taste—of, for example, chickpea falafels, hommus with whole grain pita points, bean-based soups such as minestrone, lentil, and split pea, or bean-filled burritos—acts as a foundation for the rest of a meal. Peanuts have a fan club all their own.

Some people are down on beans because, frankly, they cause gas. From "the first marine who found the bean, parlez-vous" to "beans, beans, they're good for your heart, the more you eat, the more you . . . ," many a silly rhyme relies on this fact. Yes, beans are *oligosaccharides*, which means that some of the carbohydrate, instead of being absorbed, gets passed on to the bacteria in the lower digestive tracts and ends up as flatulence. Cooking beans thoroughly and eating them slowly helps to reduce the problem.

Basically, legumes are very flexible foods. They calm and strengthen at the same time, making them "the velvet and the steel" of a high performance nutritional program. From a dietary perspective, soybeans anchor the legume family. A host of other beans add variety and flavor.

SOYBEANS

Notable Personality Factors: Although soybeans are still considered some-what exotic in the United States, they are as basic as bread in Asian cultures, and have been cultivated in such countries as China and Japan for thou-sands of years. Soy has a remarkably versatile personality. Tofu (bean curd derived from soy milk), one of the most popular renditions of soy protein, is a central component of any vegetarian diet. A sensible substitute for dairy and eggs, it can even be scrambled for breakfast. The soy milk itself is a healthy alternative to cow's milk, and is recommended for pregnant and nursing women, infants making the switch to the bottle, and the elderly. It's also an excellent energizer, and helps to add thickness and texture to fruit smoothies. Miso, a fermented soy paste, soothes the digestive and nervous systems—miso soup is renowned for its ability to calm and ground. And tem-peh, a high-protein soy product made by fermenting cooked beans, is often adopted as a meat substitute by those converting to a vegetarian diet. In fact, on first taste—as an ingredient in, for example, an Indonesian dish—tempeh is often mistaken for meat. This is partially because of its texture, which is more coarse than that of tofu or even soy burgers.

As this inventory indicates, the soybean is an incredibly adaptable legume. Do note, however, that although soy cheese provides the pleasing taste without the fat of pasteurized spreads, it should be eaten in modera-tion, no more than two or three times per week. One other exception: soy sauce. Unfortunately, soy sauce is probably the most popular soy product in the United States, but it's very high in salt and, depending on where it's served, may contain MSG. I recommend instead Liquid Aminos, which offers a similar flavor and fragrance without the excess sodium.

Therapeutic and Healing Powers: Soybeans are super-alkaline, more alka-line than any other legume. As such, they protect against all the common, over-acidic, oxidative, degenerative diseases, and can be prescribed to treat arthritis, diabetes, heart ailments, multiple sclerosis, and cancer. The low incidence of colon cancer in China and Japan has been attributed in part to the high degree of soy in the two countries' diets. And research has recently linked soybeans to the prevention of breast cancer. Isoflavones, protease inhibitors, beta-sitosterol, and other phytonutrients in soy act as anti-estro-gens. In effect, because of their estrogenic chemistry, they fool the body, thereby preventing it from overproducing the hormone itself: Soy nutrients occupy competitive estrogen binding sites and so keep a woman's own natural estrogen from binding to these same sites and inducing cancer in estrogen-sensitive tissues such as the breasts and ovaries. By the same token, phytoestrogens help to balance hormonal fluctuations that occur over the course of a woman's monthly menstrual cycle. For example, tofu sedates the mood swings associated with PMS.

The fiber content in soybeans makes enough of an impact to influence the body to lower cholesterol. Special soy phytonutrients also support the pancreas by enhancing the effectiveness of insulin. In general, soy has the ability to balance blood sugar and ward off the highs and lows of diabetes and functional hypoglycemia. Of course, soy is also a powerful protein—remember that tofu and tempeh made the top ten list of energizing foods (Chapter 10). Overall, soybeans embody the dietary ideal of preventive medicine.

Nutrient Value: Of all the legumes, soybean sprouts have the highest concentration of protein—about 40 to 50 percent. Soybeans are also high in fat (mostly unsaturated) and essential fatty acids. They offer significant amounts of calcium, iron, and potassium, and are substantial sources of vitamins E, B_6, and B_{12}, and folic acid. They contain all the essential amino acids found in meat proteins, along with phytonutrients proven to lower blood cholesterol.

Selection and Care: Soy is available in a variety of forms, be it milk in the dairy aisle, sprouts bunched alongside the leafy vegetables, or prepackaged tofu patties. Just be sure to buy quality brands from reputable health food stores.

Optimal Use and Combining: Tofu and tempeh add heft to brown rice and vegetable plates. They also add protein to pasta or potatoes. For lunch, "cottage" tofu salads or eggless tofu "egg" salads are becoming increasingly popular. Soy hot dogs and burgers are other solid protein meals. Try soy cheese on seven-grain bread and soy milk in fruit smoothies. To quell a sweet craving, whip up some tofu cheesecake. Make soy products a staple of your vegetarian entrees, and eat them about three times a week.

LENTILS

Notable Personality Factors: Lentils have an intrigue all their own. Among the first crops raised by prehistoric man, they are said to have originated in Asia, but are biblically tied to the Holy Land. Egyptians and Israelis consider

lentils to have been the central ingredient in the pottage for which Esau sold his birthright to Jacob.

A classic high-protein, high-fiber, low-fat meat substitute, lentils have a distinct personality and prefer center stage. They refuse to be relegated to the status of side dish or garnish. They demand respect. For fall and winter feasts, I recommend lentil nut roasts as a healthy, hearty alternative to turkeys and hams.

Like other legumes, lentils both stabilize and energize, nurture and stimulate the body. They're also considered brain food, and boost intelligence.

Therapeutic and Healing Powers: The lentil's remedial properties are similar to those of the soybean. Essentially, they help to prevent cancer, lower cholesterol, and balance blood sugar. For this last reason, they are recommended for diabetics and hypoglycemics. Because lentils contain a specific blend of minerals that build the blood, they are also useful in the treatment of anemia. These legumes stimulate the liver to purge the body of biochemical poisons, and they manage pancreatic-adrenal stress quite efficiently. Lentil loaves and burgers provide a concentrated serving of protein and also lubricate frazzled nerves.

Nutrient Value: In addition to consisting of nearly 30 percent protein, lentils are also packed with essential minerals. They contain calcium, copper, iron, magnesium, and potassium. And they offer a diverse supply of B vitamins.

Selection and Care: Lentils are available either canned or dried. As much as possible depending on packaging, check that the beans are free from gravel and other filler. Skins should be smooth, not wrinkled or blistered. Store lentils in a tightly sealed glass jar in a cool, dark place. (Note that these same criteria apply to selecting and storing all other beans.)

Optimal Use and Combining: Along with tofu, lentils should be a staple of any high-performance meal plan. It's best, however, not to overload on beans by combining the two. Instead of eating lentils with other legumes, pair them with potatoes or rice. They also ground a leafy green vegetable salad. From fall through spring, lentil soup hits the spot. To prepare, boil three cups of lentils in six cups of water for about an hour to an hour and a half. Simmer until the lentils are tender. Add celery, carrots, onions, mushrooms, and herbs to the brew for a savory vegetarian stew.

Get to know your legumes. Other members of the family share the same traits as the soybean and lentil, and all help to ground the metabolism and safeguard the body against erratic, destabilizing food swings. For variety, occasionally substitute soybeans or lentils with some of the following legumes. All are high in protein, low in saturated fat, and high in fiber.

Pinto Beans: Pinto beans are the basis for the classic Mexican dip and make the best tostadas and burritos. Paired with organic corn chips, they're a healthy party snack. They also season vegetarian chilis. Combine with corn and avocado to make a complete protein.

Navy or Kidney Beans: Kidney beans hail from South American, Mexican, and Native American cultures. They're probably best known as an ingredient in soup, but they can also garnish a garden salad. To enhance their flavor, combine with carrots, tomatoes, and zucchinis.

Garbonzo Beans: Also known as chickpeas, garbonzo beans are a nutritional delicacy believed to have originated in the Middle East. They can be added raw to salads, cooked and mashed into a hommus dip, or fried into crunchy falafels. For example, whole-wheat pita spread with hommus or stuffed with a falafel patty makes a solid lunchtime sandwich; falafel can also substitute for meatballs in a bowl of spaghetti.

Lima Beans: Carved out of Peruvian culture, lima beans were named after the country's capital city. Although not quite as high in protein as soybeans, lentils, or even chickpeas, lima beans are celebrated for their ability to simultaneously calm and energize. Admittedly, these beans tend to be more flagrant when it comes to flatulence. To minimize this explosive aspect of their personality, I recommend soaking the beans for one hour before cooking. Lima bean soup is another legume classic, and the beans go well with green vegetables.

Split Peas: Of all the legumes, split peas have the highest concentration of pantothenic acid, the nutrient that nurtures the adrenal glands. At 28 percent protein, they are comparable to lentils, although they are lower in calcium. Rounding out the list of legume-based soups, split pea is a cold-weather favorite. Split peas can also be tossed in leafy green salads— throw in some sesame seeds to up the protein quotient. Carrots and peas make a dynamic combo, almost nutritious enough to rival romaine lettuce. Peas also go well with mushrooms, and together they add flavor and texture to a creamy pasta dish.

CHAPTER 18

NUT AND SEED PERSONALITIES

My coverage of the personality of foods would be incomplete without a mention of nuts and seeds. Nuts and seeds add character and crunch to meals. Their natural oils keep the metabolic machinery operating smoothly. They fine-tune a high-performance diet, and they've earned a reputation as nutritional facilitators: Their enzymes, amino acids, and phytonutrients unleash the dietary powers of vegetables and fruits.

Smart food combining creates positive food swings. The idea is to team together nutritional players with opposite, complementary strengths. It's all about balance. For example, fruits are low in protein; nuts are high in protein. Combined, nuts maximize the nutrients in fruits and transform the salad into a complete protein. The same is true of seeds and vegetables: Sunflower or sesame seeds act as a catalyst, converting fresh, raw, garden salads into complete proteins. Sprouted seeds make the dish that much more nutritious.

When nuts and seeds are added to fruit and vegetable salads, a refreshing dish becomes a restorative one. If fruits and vegetables are cleansers, then nuts and seeds are "closers." They complete a meal by rounding out its protein content. And complete protein, containing all essential amino acids, is the key to sound vegetarian nutrition and peak biological performance, because protein repairs damaged tissue, generates new tissue, and energizes.

In addition to their premium protein, nuts and seeds are also packed with vitamins and minerals. Their phytoenzymatic protease inhibitors aid in the suppression of cancerous cell growth. And although they are high in fat, it's largely of the unsaturated (that is, good) kind. My top nut is the almond, and my top seed, the peanut. But familiarize yourself with the various flavors of other nuts and seeds, and experiment with different combinations in order to create superior nutrition.

ALMONDS

Notable Personality Factors: Romantic folklore surrounds almonds. Ancient symbols of fertility, to this day they are given out as favors at weddings. Their sweet, almost buttery flavor naturally lends itself to spreads. Sliced or chopped, they add texture and taste to rice dishes, whole grain cereals, and, of course, fruit salads. Almonds are considered to have come from the mild climates of northern Africa, and are associated with many classic Middle Eastern dishes, but California is currently the leading producer of the plant.

Therapeutic and Healing Powers: Like tempeh (see Chapter 17), almond butter is another excellent vegetarian alternative to meat protein. As such, it helps to manage and ultimately correct functional hypoglycemia, ease digestive disorders, and bulk up muscles. Moreover, almond butter on seven-grain bread acts as a dietary aphrodisiac (on rice cakes, it's just as nutritious, if not as sensual). Almonds are quite alkaline, and pair well with equally alkaline watermelon. They can alleviate rheumatism, adjust body fluids, and fortify the immune system. And they help to regulate the thyroid and adrenal glands. For its calcium, I recommend almond-sesame milk to pregnant or nursing women. Of course, it can also be used by anyone in cereal or smoothies.

Almonds contain amygdalin, also known as laetrile, which is considered a protease-inhibiting anti-cancerous ingredient. (The laetrile cancer cure spread through Mexico and southern California some twenty-five years ago.) The high arginine content in the nut can, however, aggravate herpes.

Nutrient Value: Almonds are about 20 percent protein and more than 50 percent fat. They contain a unique blend of magnesium, potassium, and zinc, and are second only to sesame seeds in their calcium concentration. They also supply vitamins B and E.

Selection and Care: Store almonds in airtight containers and refrigerate for crispness.

Optimal Use and Combining: Toss almonds in fresh, alkaline fruit salads—try them out with watermelon, honeydew, papaya, and cantaloupe. Spread almond butter on whole grain breads. Almonds mix well with cashews and sunflower seeds, as well as with wheat in crunchy granolas.

PEANUTS

Notable Personality Factors: Mmmmm, peanuts. Another American classic. Peanut butter and jelly sandwiches, peanuts and Cracker Jacks at the ballpark, packets of peanuts on the airplane—we're nuts about these seeds! In fact, even though they originated in South America, peanuts are now a prevalent crop in the United States. Peanut butter in particular is often associated with childhood, and for this reason is often a mommy-daddy food. When salted, covered in chocolate, or sprinkled on top of ice cream sundaes, the negatives overwhelm the positives in peanuts. Instead, skip the sugary coatings and stick with dry-roasted, unsalted, unhydrogenated peanuts and peanut butter. In their pure form, peanuts provide protein and energy. Peanut butter is similar to almond butter in its actions. It's soothing, grounding, tenacious.

Recently, peanuts have come under fire, accused of containing a carcinogen. Specifically, peanuts are susceptible to the growth of a fungus that can produce aflatoxin, a cancer-causing agent. Raw peanuts present the most risk: The high temperatures of the dry-roasting process inactivate the aflatoxin. That's why I prefer peanut butter to whole, raw peanuts.

Therapeutic and Healing Powers: I prescribe peanut butter to patients who need to increase the protein in their diets. Like almond butter, it can cure burnout and low blood sugar.

Nutrient Value: Peanuts have a higher protein content than any other commonplace nut or seed, even almonds. They also have a lower percentage of fat. Peanuts are rich in B vitamins and such minerals as magnesium.

Selection and Care: The same as for almonds.

Optimal Use and Combining: Peanuts combine better with acid fruits than do almonds. For example, they mix well with berries. They also add their distinctive flavor to whole wheat breads and certain Middle Eastern-influenced rice dishes. With a few exceptions, they don't usually pair well with vegetables. Peanut oil is high in polyunsaturated fat, which converts into trans-fatty acids when heated, so it's still better to use olive oil when cooking.

Other members of the nut family have similar beneficial properties as almonds. They support fruits, facilitate nutritional balance, close out complete proteins, lubricate organs and tissues, and stabilize metabolic systems. In addition to almonds, other popular nuts include:

Cashews: Cashews have a very distinct, perfumed flavor that combines well with almost all types of fruit. They're lower in fat than most other nuts, but also lower in calcium and vitamin E. In addition to a typically high protein content, cashews also contain significant amounts of iron and zinc. Cashew food stuffs include milk and butter, both of which can occasionally take the place of their almond equivalents.

Walnuts: Virile and meaty, walnuts add rich taste and texture to granolas, soups, pastas, and lentil loaves—just add mushroom gravy and call it a day. In terms of fruit partnering, they prefer acid to alkaline varieties. Walnuts are full of minerals and vitamin E.

Brazil Nuts: Brazil nuts are high in methionine, making them an excellent match for legumes, which are usually low in the amino acid. They're also high in saturated fat, second only to the coconut.

As for seeds, jack up the protein content of vegetable dishes by incorporating any of these scrumptious options:

Sunflower Seeds: Like nuts, sunflower seeds are nurturing and restorative, with a high percentage of protein. Many Americans are addicted to the seeds in their salted shells but, of course, this is not the healthiest snack. Instead, stay away from the salt, and add unshelled seeds to raw vegetable salads. Stocked with phytoenzymes, sunflower seed sprouts are also super-alkaline, and belong in the salads of anyone at risk for or suffering from cancer. High in calcium, iron, and other minerals, sunflower seeds supply essential fatty acids that oil the system, lower cholesterol, and reduce blood pressure. Sunflower seed dip brings robust flavor to organic chips and whole wheat bread.

Sesame Seeds: These diverse, adaptable seeds, teeming with methionine, combine well with tofu, lentils, and garbonzo beans to form complete proteins.

In the form of almond-sesame milk, their calcium makes them a perfect substitute for dairy. Toss hulled seeds in raw vegetable salads and profit from the antioxidants and protease inhibitors.

Pumpkin Seeds: Not just for Halloween! Pumpkin seeds can be eaten soft, fresh, and raw or dry-roasted (no salt). In addition to their high protein and oil content, they supply healthy doses of zinc, and that makes them a valuable nutritional tool in the prevention of prostate disorders. Their mineral concentration has also gained them a reputation as fertility enhancers. As with other seeds, include pumpkin seeds in fresh vegetable salads.

Flaxseed: Brimming with linoleic and omega-3 fatty acids, flaxseed oil protects against coronary disease, high cholesterol, and stroke. One to two tablespoons of cold-processed flaxseed oil also acts as an anti-inflammatory aid, and is reputed to treat such autoimmune disorders as lupus and multiple sclerosis.

RESOURCE

F **or further information** or to order Re-Vita:

Re-Vita
153 Industrial Loop South
Orange Park, FL 32073
(800) 442-7005
www.re-vita.net

ABOUT THE AUTHOR

Barnet Meltzer, M.D. has been a board certified physician and surgeon for over twenty-five years and was the first medical doctor to enter the clinical practice of Preventative Medicine in southern California. He currently has a private practice in Del Mar, California, through which he has helped thousands of people sustain vitality and energize their lifestyles with his Wellness Program. Dr. Meltzer is the author of several books, including *The Complete 21-Day Del Mar Diet* and *The Ten Laws of High Performance Wellness*. He and his family live in Del Mar, California.